Group Work with the Emotionally Disabled

The *Social Work with Groups* series

Series Editors: Catherine P. Papell and Beulah Rothman

- *Co-Leadership in Social Work with Groups*, Catherine P. Papell and Beulah Rothman
- *Social Groupwork & Alcoholism*, Marjorie Altman and Ruth Crocker, Guest Editors
- *Groupwork with the Frail Elderly*, Shura Saul, Guest Editor
- *The Use of Group Services in Permanency Planning for Children*, Sylvia Morris, Guest Editor
- *Activities and Action in Groupwork*, Ruth Middleman, Guest Editor
- *Groupwork with Women/Groupwork with Men: An Overview of Gender Issues in Social Groupwork Practice*, Beth Glover Reed and Charles D. Garvin, Guest Editors
- *Ethnicity in Social Group Work Practice*, Larry Davis, Guest Editor
- *Groupwork with Children and Adolescents*, Ralph Kolodny and James Garland, Guest Editors
- *Time as a Factor in Groupwork*, Albert Alissi and Max Casper, Guest Editors
- *The Legacy of William Schwartz: Group Practice as Shared Interaction*, Alex Gitterman and Lawrence Shulman, Guest Editors
- *Research in Social Group Work*, Sheldon D. Rose and Ronald A. Feldman, Guest Editors
- *Collectivity in Social Group Work: Concept and Practice*, Norma C. Lang and Joanne Sulman, Guest Editors
- *Working Effectively with Administrative Groups*, Ronald W. Toseland and Paul H. Ephross, Guest Editors
- *Violence: Prevention and Treatment in Groups*, George S. Getzel, Guest Editor
- *Group Work with the Poor and Oppressed*, Judith A. G. Lee, Guest Editor
- *Social Work with Multi-Family Groups*, D. Rosemary Cassano, Guest Editor
- *Groups in Health Care Settings*, Janice H. Schopler and Maeda J. Galinsky, Guest Editors
- *Group Work with the Emotionally Disabled*, Baruch Levine, Guest Editor

Group Work with the Emotionally Disabled

Baruch Levine
Editor

Routledge
Taylor & Francis Group
New York London

Routledge is an imprint of the
Taylor & Francis Group, an informa business

Group Work with the Emotionally Disabled has also been published as *Social Work with Groups*, Volume 13, Number 1 1990.

Reprinted 2009 by Routledge

Library of Congress Cataloging-in-Publication Data

Group work with the emotionally disabled / Baruch Levine, guest editor.
p. cm.
"Also published as Social work with groups, volume 13, number 1, 1990"–T.p. verso.
Includes bibliographical references.
ISBN 0-86656-994-4
1. Group psychotherapy. 2. Social group work. I. Levine, Baruch. II. Social work with groups (Haworth Press)
RC488.G744 1990
616.89'152–dc20 90-4281
CIP

Group Work with the Emotionally Disabled

CONTENTS

ABOUT THE EDITOR

Baruch Levine, PhD, maintains a private practice, counseling groups, individuals, and families. He is also a half-time associate professor at the Jane Addams College of Social Work, University of Illinois at Chicago. Dr. Levine has had many years of experience in the psychiatric field, pioneering both the combination of teaching group work and casework and the development of milieu therapy. He has had extensive consultation experience in the use of groups for a wide variety of social work endeavors including child welfare and guidance, medical social work, family service, corrections, and aging. Recently, he has been concentrating his activities on services to minorities, alcoholics, and the homeless. Dr. Levine is the author of *Fundamentals of Group Treatment* (Whitehall, 1967), *Group Psychotherapy: Practice and Development* (Prentice-Hall, 1979), and with Virginia Gallogly, *Group Therapy with Alcoholics* (Sage, 1985).

Group Work with the Emotionally Disabled

Preface

The coexistence of mental illness and mental health in effective group experiences for treating mental disability is the message of this volume edited by Baruch Levine. Levine, a prestigious social group worker and clinical theorist, points out that historically, in its insistence on supporting and reaching for strength, social group work may have been less attuned to illness. Retrospectively, had social group work been less fearful that by identifying itself with psychotherapy its commitment to the healthy aspects of human functioning would be obscured, the richness of its techniques and approaches for the treatment of the mentally ill might have earlier been recognized. Levine hypothesizes that by viewing social group work as a field of practice with group psychotherapy as one of many methods, in this case a specific social work method for treating the mentally ill in groups, the balance in perceiving and simultaneously dealing with the duality of illness and strength might more readily be maintained. This is an intriguing conceptualization for the profession of social work and it invites continuing discussion.

Baruch Levine's landmark book, *Group Psychotherapy* (Englewood Cliffs, N.J.: Prentice-Hall, Inc., 1979), is an important resource where can be found a dynamic integration of group psychotherapy and social group work. Now in this collection of papers on social group work practice with the emotionally disabled, which Levine edits, our readers are provided with a history of the development of its use in psychiatric settings. Inviting Gisela Konopka and John Wax, both participants and presenters in the first conference on Group Work in Psychiatric Settings (1957), was a creative editorial act. The past and future perspectives, along with the excellent practice papers selected for this volume, reveal how far we have come.

The fine line between understanding the depth of illness and the potential of wellness is captured, as we could well expect by our revered social group work colleague, Gisela Konopka. Accepting the vulnerability of the mentally ill along with the intrinsic strengths of the human condition, Konopka calls for "the gentle use of the positive aspects of group process and the goal of enhancement of the individual's power and capacity."

We come full circle with John Wax's affirmation that now, as then, the essential characteristic of social group work is helping people develop and use resources, and, says Wax, "resources are the real stuff of staying out of psychiatric hospitals."

While social group work recognizes that it has often been admonished for inattention to the deeply internal individualistic aspects of dysfunction, the papers chosen for presentation in this volume suggest that in a contemporary light the special focus of the social group work methodology seems to have much to offer to the new approaches to the treatment of mental illness. As pointed out by Bond and De Graaf-Kaser, research findings indicate that group approaches emphasizing the normal human and developmental needs of the mentally ill, treatment in natural settings and structured skills development are essential ingredients of effective treatment. Contemporary group treatment modalities employed by other disciplines seem to have adopted many of the goals and practice principles familiar and fundamental to the social group worker.

The social group work practice papers selected by the editor and his advisory committee for this volume illuminate the versatility, knowledge and skill of Baruch Levine's standards of excellence. They also demonstrate the traditional values and creative use of resources suggested by Konopka and Wax.

The settings for group treatment of the chronically ill and psychiatrically at-risk run the gamut from community (Rose) and school (Schamess), out-patient forensic clinic (Gamblin), in-patient psychiatric unit (Armstrong), continuing care clinic (DiDemenico), and finally a maximum security hospital (Wolozin and Dalton).

The practice papers reveal a concensus regarding the primacy of group processes that has been present in social group work since its earliest days. Group cohesion in working with the emotionally disabled is a requirement for achieving any treatment goal. Rose, in discussing the group treatment of agoraphobia, points to the power of the group as a reinforcer when it is characterized by "cooperation, internal interpersonal liking, attraction to the leader, and concern for others." The paper by Rose is a lucid group treatment scenario for persons with agoraphobia. His commitment to making knowledge available for replication and further validation is evident. To be seen repeatedly is the ever-present use of activity and program developed in creative ways through exercises, assignments, rituals—all experiential means by which the purposes of the group are fostered.

The practitioner authors are in step with current conceptualizations and theoretical orientations that are available for therapeutic use. They are creative in making use of new ideas, formulations and skills without loss of the rootedness in the major premises of social group work. While recognizing internal conflict and emotional states of the members there is a universal commitment to staying with mastery of socialization and everyday living skills.

There is universal conviction that group processes not be used to stimulate or incite the expression of irrational and negative behavior. While feelings are accepted, recognized and discussed the strength of the group, with the help of the worker, to support healthy containment in the interest of growth in social functioning is ever present.

We congratulate Baruch Levine for developing an exciting and informative volume. It identifies social group work's roots in the treatment of emotionally disabled persons. It affirms the significance of social group work's clinical potential and it propels us to further development in this highly specialized area of human service.

CP
BR

Acknowledgements

Many thanks to the following people for their help in the development of this edition: Stephen Z. Cohen, PhD, Associate Professor at the Jane Addams College of Social Work of the University of Illinois at Chicago; Virginia Gallogly, MSW, LCSW, private practitioner in Chicago, Illinois; and Richard Tolman, PhD, Assistant Professor at the Jane Addams College of Social Work of the University of Illinois at Chicago.

PAST/PRESENT ISSUES IN GROUP WORK WITH THE EMOTIONALLY DISABLED

Thirty-Five Years of Group Work in Psychiatric Settings

This volume is dedicated to the 35th anniversary of the first conference on Group Work in Psychiatric Settings. In his paper, Baruch Levine, editor of this volume, elaborates on some of the problems and issues in group work with the emotionally disabled raised at the 1950s conferences. These issues continue to plague education for group work with the emotionally disabled today. As part of this editorial we are also fortunate to have updates from two of the participants in the early conferences on psychiatric group work.

Gisela Konopka (1956), professor and director emeritus of the University of Minnesota School of Social Work, pioneered the development of group work in psychiatric settings and served as the keynote speaker in the first conference, GROUP WORK IN THE PSYCHIATRIC SETTING held at Shades Inn Park in Waveland, Indiana on June 27 to July 2, 1955, and funded by the National Institute of Mental Health. Professor Konopka elaborates on how the enabling and freeing powers of social group work are often lost in some current tendencies toward the use of groups for subjugation and conformity in psychiatric settings.

John Wax (1960), chief social worker of the Veteran's Administration Hospital in Palo Alto California and one of the early social work practitioners with groups in psychiatric settings, delivered a paper in another of the early conferences, USE OF GROUPS IN THE PSYCHIATRIC SETTING held at the Kellog Center for Continuing Education in East Lansing, Michigan on June 13 to 16, 1958 and funded by the National Institute of Mental Health. Mr. Wax connects the use of groups in psychiatric settings to social work through consideration of the common goal of empowering members to use their inner and outer resources.

Part I

Baruch Levine

Group work with the emotionally disabled began in the post war period. However, most of the work was being accomplished by psychiatric social workers who were trained primarily to work with individuals. Gisela Konopka, in a paper delivered at the Dartmouth Conference on Education for Psychiatric Social Work in 1949, called attention to the need for graduate schools of social work to provide training in group work for the psychiatric social workers.

Group work education in graduate schools of social work was first introduced at the School of Applied Social Sciences of Western Reserve University in Cleveland, Ohio in 1923. In 1934 the New York School of Social Work of Columbia University and in 1938 The Pittsburgh University School of Social Work introduced group work as part of the social work curriculum. During the 40s group work education spread through the graduate schools of social work (Coyle 1960).

Early group work was focused on primary community settings such as settlement houses and community centers. The major concern was the disadvantaged. Most of the work was done with children and adolescents and their families. As a direct consequence, most of the people teaching group work were experienced in working with the disadvantaged and they were not necessarily familiar with direct work with emotionally disabled.

In June of 1955 a conference on Group Work in the Psychiatric Setting (Trecker 1956), sponsored by the American Association of Group Workers and funded by the National Institute of Mental Health, was held to focus on the development of theory and application of group work methods to the field of mental health. A second conference entitled, Use of Groups in the Psychiatric Setting, sponsored by the National Association of Social Workers (1960), was held three years later in June of 1958. These two conferences brought together many of the group workers and case workers who were pioneering the use of group techniques with the emotionally disabled.

As a neophyte to group work and particularly psychiatric group work around the time of these conferences, the ideas formulated in the proceedings served as early guidelines for my work in applying group work knowledge and techniques to psychiatric settings. What I found most interesting in returning to some of these early codifications of psychiatric group work knowledge is that many of the same issues that were raised at these conferences are still plaguing social group work and particularly social workers' use of groups with the emotionally disabled.

In my thirty-four years as a professional group worker, much of which was in working with and teaching about use of groups with the emotionally disabled, I have had to live with the issues raised in those early conferences and would like to offer some possible insights into why these dilemmas remain and what might be done about them.

GROUP WORK – GROUP THERAPY

One of the early issues social workers faced as they entered psychiatric settings was concern about group work and group therapy becoming confused (Konopka 1956). The fear was that a certain prestige might be attached to group therapy and cause social workers in other settings to be in awe or envy of psychiatric group work. This fear was felt even earlier as between generic casework and psychiatric casework. While I and many other early psychiatric group workers held to social group work being something different from group therapy, other disciplines often picked up group work techniques and called it group therapy.

The problem is that all disciplines on the psychiatric team have become interested in groups and are less concerned with what it is called and more concerned with what kind of group work helps. As a consequence, mainly psychologists and some psychiatrists, with much less organized background and theory about groups were soon regarded as the group therapy experts. Often these people knew a great deal more about individual psychodynamics but much less about groups. Nevertheless, if a group was called therapy then psychologists or psychiatrists were often sought out for supervision. One psychologist that I knew received his early group experiences as a student volunteer in a group work agency. Very soon after he became a psychologist he was considered a group therapy expert and was supervising social workers and others on their work with groups.

The concern about group therapy in social group work appeared to arise from two major sources. First is the general trend in social work education and among social work educators to abhor the idea of social workers doing psychotherapy. This abhorrence arose during the time psychoanalysis had a firm grip on the whole treatment field. Certainly, a master's degree social work education did not prepare one to do psychoanalytic treatment. However, the general trend toward ego psychology and a wider variety of individual and family treatment approaches makes the overlap with social work even more diffuse. The increased focus on the individual and family and the individual and environment in the mental health field further obfuscate the distinctions between social work and other disciplines. It almost seems as if the rest of the psychiatric field moved toward social work approaches to treatment, making distinctions increasingly difficult.

The other problem was that most social group work educators had little or no background in psychiatric group work and could not teach from their experiences. As a result they would concentrate on more generic group work based on experiences in social group work agencies. These experiences were with primarily normal or slightly problemed children and teenagers compared to the psychiatric group workers who had to primarily work with seriously problemed adults. Many of these educators, even today, teach basic group work skills and may introduce group therapy as developed by psychologists or psychiatrists. Some have told me that they won't use a book on group therapy written by a social worker because it presents a bad model. What they are saying is that because of their bias against the word psychotherapy they are not going to use material that might synthesize group work and group therapy for social workers. After graduation, most social workers in treatment settings are required to do group therapy and have to seek training. If these social workers were taught that group therapy is not in the province of social work, they must look to psychologists and psychiatrists for that training. The result is that while group work, in the author's opinion, has a more coherent theoretical framework for group treatment, social work practitioners become more reliant on theories from other disciplines that are less well developed.

Group work has much to offer and has made a large contribution to the field of group psychotherapy. Due to the overlap of techniques and function in the current work with the emotionally disabled, it is puzzling why we dwell on the distinctions between group work and group psychotherapy. Why not prepare social work students to value their social work contributions and relate it to what they will be called upon to practice in the real world? Might it also help the growth of generic group work to incorporate new developments in group therapy in social work education?

Konopka and Wax, in their respective contributions to this article, aptly point to basic values and functions that social workers can bring to work with the emotionally disabled. Do social workers lose sight of these values and functions if they are not imbued with a social work perspective on group therapy?

GENERIC GROUP WORK – PSYCHIATRIC GROUP WORK

In her keynote paper at the 1955 conference, "The Generic and the Specific in Group Work Practice in the Psychiatric Setting," Konopka (1956) profoundly points out the bases of group work practice that might support practice in any setting. She points to the values, knowledge and methods to which a group worker would easily subscribe.

Konopka (1956) also points to some of the specific differences that might characterize psychiatric group work.

1. Intensified individualization . . .
2. An especially high skill in and focus on formation of groups . . .
3. Skill in dealing with emotionally charged verbal material . . .
4. More acquaintance with medical and psychiatric knowledge . . .

5. Capacity to accept and know other professions and yet keep one's own identity and be able to interpret it to others.
6. Capacity to accept mental and emotional illness and work with it.

She further suggests that these specifics might appear in other aspects of practice but are especially necessary in psychiatric settings.

Konopka's development of the generic and specific aspects of group work in psychiatric settings has persisted over the years. However, there are some distinctions that are less achievable theoretically. These arise from the differences in group work practice in primary agencies and special settings.

Group work in primary agencies was more a field of practice than a method of practice. Although there was much work with groups in primary agencies, group workers and group work agencies were involved in a myriad of other services. Informal education, health and welfare services were the major functions. Group work agencies arose to help resettle the many immigrants to the cities both from foreign countries and rural parts of the United States. Work with groups derived from the informal education services provided by these community agencies. Even today, work with groups is not a major part of the services provided by these agencies. It appears that informal education, casework, community organization and advocacy are the major methods employed in group work agencies today.

Group work agencies began with the goals of helping in the adjustment of newcomers to the cities, the uplifting and enhancement of the disadvantaged in the cities and working for social change. At different times, in accordance with changing needs, group work agencies have emphasized different combinations of these goals.

Work with the emotionally disabled brought very different kinds of goals. Social adjustment and improving function were primary foci. In his paper at the 1958 conference, Raymond Fisher pointed out how psychiatric social workers conducting groups were much more familiar with the needs and kinds of help that psychiatric clients required (Fisher 1960). Group workers from traditional agencies were not familiar with these needs and ways of helping. Instead, Fisher questioned the transposition of traditional group work techniques to psychiatric settings rather than adaptation of the techniques to suit the new demands.

Fisher (1960) posited the relationship of

group work – group treatment – casework

as the province of neither specialty. He further suggested that group workers needed to learn much more about helping the mentally ill while caseworkers needed to learn more about groups in order to do group treatment.

Group workers had training and experience with group methods while caseworkers had experience with the goals of helping psychiatric patients. Was background with group work more important than background in casework with psychiatric patients or vice versa? Since most social work educators in those early days of group treatment had experience in either casework with emotionally disabled or group work in primary agencies, the question became which background was more important for teaching group treatment. Was knowledge of the group method more important than knowledge of helping psychiatric clients or vice versa? In most instances the option taken was familiarity with the method rather than familiarity with the goals. As a result, group work was most often taught by faculty who had a background in traditional group work and little or no familiarity with use of groups with the emotionally disabled.

Another problem that besets the training of group workers for the emotionally disabled arises from the unevenness in the development of traditional group work and treatment in groups. Traditional group work was and is accomplished through the work of volunteers, part time staff, or group work students. Very little direct service to groups was accomplished by professional group workers. The net result of this situation was that the highest level of group work skill realized in primary group work settings was that of second year students or recent graduates. While professional group workers supervised the practice, they couldn't achieve the level of practice that they might if they continued to work directly with groups themselves.

Group work in psychiatric settings was and is generally accomplished by trained professionals who bring their knowledge and skills into the treatment session and do not continuously work through less or untrained assistants. The level of knowledge and skill developed from professional direct practice is bound to surpass that of group work in primary settings. As a result, it would be difficult for teachers of group work who have never experienced more sophisticated practice to qualitatively impart that knowledge and skill.

GROUP WORK AND THE TEACHING OF INTEGRATED METHODS

While groups are employed more than ever in psychiatric settings, there appears to be less and less interest in group work education in schools of social work. This disinterest in the schools of social work is paralleled by less interest on the part of students and professional workers in obtaining training in group from schools of social work.

One of the major factors that appears to influence this phenomenon is the burgeoning popularity of family treatment. Family methods appear to be enjoying the kind of popularity that group methods enjoyed in the 1960s and 70s.

Another possible reason for the lessening of interest in group work is that there is little conviction of the efficacy of group treatment by most teachers of social work methods. Teaching individual, family and group work in one synthesized course might best be accomplished by someone who has had training and experience in all three methods. While there are some educators who have had all three experiences, most have not. Even those who have had all three experiences might have emphasized one or two and have dabbled in the others. The result is that they might have little or no conviction about the efficacy of the methods in which they have not really invested. Aside from the theoretical discussion of methodology, students do get a feeling from the teacher about what is really important and helpful and what may be interesting but less consequential for helping people.

Most teachers of integrated methods have had training and experience in individual treatment and, increasingly, many have also had training and experience in family treatment. Few have had training and any significant experience in group treatment. As a result, group treatment receives low priority in most teaching of integrated methods. While some of the teachers of integrated methods are group workers, most of whom have never had a treatment group experience, there is little transmission of conviction about the efficacy of groups for treatment. At best, group treatment is taught as an interesting method to be employed for objectives that are ancillary to the real work to be done.

CONCLUSIONS

Some of the very problems and issues cited by Konopka and Fisher in those early conferences on group work in psychiatric settings are still with us. The fear of group therapy still abounds and affects not only the education for psychiatric settings, but the limiting of substance for full partnership of group work in education for generic treatment.

One possible answer to the problem is to recognize that group work is both a field and a method. Perhaps a separation of the field and the method might allow both to grow and flourish.

The group work field is much broader in nature and scope than the group method. Group workers in todays primary agencies need a broad range of skills beyond the work with groups. Work with groups is only one of many skills like informal education, casework, family work, program planning, advocating, supervision, teaching, community organizing and administration that group workers need in order to function in the current group work field. In this current trend toward specialization in social work education, preparation for work in primary group work agencies can become one of the specialties (Lipschutz).

Group work as a pure method can then be free of some of the strictures arising from its use in a particular field and broadened into more of a generic practice method. Rather than be taught from the standpoint of traditional group work practice, teaching with treatment goals as the base of practice might help work with groups become a full partner in the teaching and learning of integrated methods.

The generics of social work practice with groups, and the rich knowledge base of group work practice might become more useful for both the social group work field and the group treatment method once the distinctions between the group work field and group method are clarified.

REFERENCES

Harleigh B. Trecker, (ed) GROUP WORK IN THE PSYCHIATRIC SETTING New York· Whiteside Inc. 1956.

USE OF GROUPS IN THE PSYCHIATRIC SETTING New York National Association of Social Workers, 1960.

Gisela Konopka "The Generic and the Specific in Group Work Practice in the Psychiatric Setting" in GROUP WORK IN THE PSYCHIATRIC SETTING op. cit. pp 11-27.

Grace Coyle "Group Work in Psychiatric Settings Its Roots and Branches" in USE OF GROUPS IN THE PSYCHIATRIC SETTING op. cit. pp. 12-22.

Raymond Fisher "Use of Groups in Social Treatment by Caseworkers and Group Workers" in USE OF GROUPS IN THE PSYCHIATRIC SETTING op. cit. pp. 23-33.

Clarence Lipschutz, a valued associate and fellow group work teacher at the University of Illinois, helped me develop the idea of separating practice with groups from group work as a field of practice.

John Wax "Criteria for Grouping Hospitalized Mental Patients" in USE OF GROUPS IN THE PSYCHIATRIC SETTING op. cit. pp 87 92.

Part II

Gisela Konopka

In 1955—over 30 years ago!—I started my discussion on group work in psychiatric settings with a quote from Walter Reed, "The prayer that has been mine for twenty years that I might be permitted in some way or at some time to do something to alleviate human suffering has been granted. A thousand happy New Years . . ."

I hoped that a thoughtful, careful, compassionate use of the group work method would help to partially fulfill such prayer for me.

Group work had special meaning to me. I had come out of the atrocious experience of Nazi Germany and searched for the best way to help people in pain, especially those who were helpless. Group work's underlying philosophy of the intense respect for the individual combined with an understanding of the power—positive and negative—of the group seemed to me a great advance in understanding of human relations and being a significantly helpful way of working with distraught and powerless people.

One-to-one work was important but group work added the ingredients of mutual help, of learning to participate in one's own fate and of not being totally in the power of the therapist alone. Ray Fisher pointed out another strength of the group work method, namely that it would allow an opportunity to "relive" as well as to "rethink."

The worth of the individual was enhanced by the group members feeling their own strength and trying them out in the presence of others "in the same boat" as well as a helpful and skilled therapist.

At the time we started talking about the use of groups in the

Gisela Konopka is Professor and Director Emeritus, University of Minnesota School of Social Work.

helping process, many professionals perceived it as an inferior way of dealing with clients.

What has happened in the last 25 years? Groups abound with emotionally upset people, children and adults. Groups have become popular vehicles for treatment, but rarely are they the kind of groups envisioned by us who underlined the basic grounding in a philosophy of respect for the individual, the skillful and gentle use of the positive aspects of group process and the goal of enhancement of the individual's power and capacity.

Groups are now frequently boring and suppressing. They are conducted by people with a need for power who make members feel attacked, who encourage mutual attack.

The power of the group process is used to enhance conformity, subjugation. Dissenters are chided, laughed at and yelled at. (This is called "confrontation.")

Sometimes groups are simply didactic pronunciations of a group leader in front of a group of clients or patients.

Other groups are one-to-one treatments with the rest of the group acting only as bystanders.

In mental hospitals for adolescents I observed groups—conducted in locked wards—where members are forced to "reveal" themselves and punished if they refuse. The marvelous intent of social group work to help people to free themselves—from their own as well as others' coercion—is lost.

The profession of social work as a whole—there are exceptions—has never recognized the great value in the development of a method that truly tried to translate social work philosophy into careful, professional practice. Many schools of social work have dropped the education for skilled group work. They also have accepted underlying philosophies alien to its great promise and thus created technicians who mechanically follow certain rules.

I hope though that some day we will revive the social group work that translated conscience into action and treated each patient with utmost respect.

I like to repeat the ending of my 1955 article which I borrowed from Eric Erickson:

> Only in so far as our clinical way of work becomes part of a judicious way of life can we help to counteract and reintegrate the destructive forces which are being let loose by the split in modern man's archaic conscience. Judiciousness in its widest sense is a frame of mind which is tolerant of differences, cautious and methodical in evaluation, just in judgment, circumspect in action and—in spite of all this apparent relativism—capable of faith and indignation.
>
> —Eric H. Erickson
> *Childhood and Society*
> (New York: W. W. Norton & Co., 1950, p. 371)

Let us keep our faith and indignation.

Part III

John Wax

As hospital psychiatry has become increasingly biological, psychologists, social workers, and to a lesser extent, nurses provide most of the day to day leadership of groups. Social workers appear to have the strongest and most coherent theoretical framework. This theoretical framework represents the congruence of therapeutic community, self help, skill building and resource development concepts.

The therapeutic community makes powerful and still novel assumptions about a psychiatric ward. Traditional psychiatry has viewed the ward as a subdivision of the hospital defined geographically as in "2 east," numerically as in "thirty beds," and diagnostically as in "female alcohol treatment." The therapeutic community sees the ward not as a location but as a social organism, an active influential environment which shapes beliefs and behaviors and which deals head on with the issue of role deprivation. The standard ward offers the patient the patient role. The therapeutic community which does almost all of its work in groups offers numerous roles: chairman of the patient council, team leader, coffee boss, treasurer of patient fund, etc. These prosocial roles must be learned and practiced and their utility for the "outside" stressed. All of these roles require skills (skill building is by far the most important goal of social work led groups). Some patients learn to handle disinfectants others learn to handle money. All of them learn to be part of a group, indeed many groups from the ward meeting for all patients and staff to the three person finance committee.

John Wax is Chief of Social Service, Veteran's Administration Hospital, Palo Alto, CA.

They learn to talk, to listen, to influence, to participate in decision making and to see that all decisions have consequences.

One of the most important beliefs in most therapeutic communities is that the individual is personally responsible for his/her own behavior and must also assume partial responsibility for the success and well being of the social system or group. This theme of personal and social responsibility is at the heart of most alcohol and other addiction programs. A variety of confrontation techniques await the patient who drinks and then tries to externalize the cause.

A variation of the personal and social responsibility ethos of the therapeutic community is the self help group which destigmatizes the problem around which the group is formed and provides helping, teaching and leadership roles. "I went from being a nobody to being a somebody." Self help groups provide powerful emotional support, shared wisdom, problem solving skills and entry into various networks. Hospital self help groups put great emphasis on plugging into counterparts in the community and preserving the bonding skills developed in the hospital.

Skill building groups appear in many forms. Discharge planning groups focus on such issues as finding housing, managing money, work transportation and recreation. They also deal with interpersonal issues such as how to deal with a room mate who smokes, a parent who is controlling or a spouse who is still abusing alcohol. Other skill building groups concentrate on how to handle the expectation that you drink, or how to cope with racist or sexist remarks. Some groups concentrate on the personal emotional and cognitive processes, i.e., How can I get control of my anger before it builds and erupts? How can I check to see if my thoughts about the board and care operator are in the ballpark with other people's thoughts? How can I get control of thoughts that keep crowding out my other thoughts? Skill building groups run the gamut from the most environmental problems to the most internal psychological processes.

A new combination of goals is addressed in the increasingly popular psycho-education groups. These groups start out as classes in a fairly formal educational format with information delivery on medications, smoking cessation, managing conflict, relapse prevention, etc. After the informational part of the meeting during which there is little discussion, the group shifts into free wheeling and quite intense discussion about problems with getting a patient to take his medication, or how to give up old drinking buddies, how to act and feel like "normal" people. In these discussions many psychotherapeutic techniques are visible – support, clarification, patterning, etc. These interventions are recommended with the knowledge objectives of the group.

Social work led groups in psychiatric hospitals are similar to social work led groups in other settings. They are about helping people identify, develop and use resources. The resource may be general assistance, ego strengths, a brother, or a mantra used to offset thoughts about having a drink. Resources are the real stuff of social work practice and resources are the real stuff of getting out of and staying out of psychiatric hospitals.

Group Approaches for Persons with Severe Mental Illness: A Typology

Gary R. Bond
Rebecca De Graaf-Kaser

SUMMARY. The development of comprehensive approaches to the treatment and rehabilitation of persons with severe mental illness has influenced the conceptualization and practice of group therapy with this population. We present a typology of group approaches, based on the dimensions of structure and locus of intervention Structure refers to the presence or absence of a defined curriculum, and locus of intervention refers to where treatment is provided. Education groups, group skills training, and some group residential models are more structured than traditional therapies, whereas psychosocial rehabilitation centers, drop-in centers, and self-help groups are more integrated with the natural environment. We discuss the advantages and disadvantages of the various approaches and implications for training and research.

Our purpose in this paper is to re-examine an old topic. the advantages and disadvantages of groups in the rehabilitation and psychological treatment of persons with severe mental illness. Our focus is limited to clients classified as "chronically mentally ill," as determined by their diagnosis (typically schizophrenia or major affective disorder), disability (role limitations in such areas as independent living and employment), and duration of illness (typically documented by at least one psychiatric hospitalization) (Goldman, Gattozzi, & Taube, 1981). The reader may wonder why still an-

---

Gary R. Bond is Associate Professor in the Department of Psychology, Indiana University-Purdue University at Indianapolis. Rebecca De Graaf-Kaser is a doctoral student in the counseling psychology program at Loyola University in Chicago. The authors express thanks to John McGrew for his suggestions on this paper.

other summary article is necessary, given reviews by Kanas (1986), Luborsky, Singer, and Luborsky (1975), Mosher and Keith (1980), Parloff and Dies (1977), and Scott and Griffith (1982). The reason is that none of these reviews have integrated the dramatic changes in the philosophy of mental health services evident in the last decade. Within the professions of social work, psychiatry, and psychology, psychotherapy and counseling have always been regarded as the basic paradigm in which psychological services are delivered. None of these professions have assimilated the concepts from psychosocial rehabilitation (PSR) (Dincin, 1975) or the Community Support Program (CSP) of the National Institute of Mental Illness (NIMH) (Stroul, 1986; Turner & TenHoor, 1978). Within the public mental health sector, however, these models are now major influences shaping program planning (Stroul, 1989).

The historical reasons for reliance on groups in mental health centers include beliefs that: (a) groups are uniquely suited to helping clients improve interpersonal skills; (b) intensive dyadic approaches are either unproductive or counterproductive for persons with severe mental illness; (c) groups are cost-effective by maximizing therapist contact time. A fourth factor explaining the popularity of groups is the recognition that medications do not remediate clients' psychosocial deficits. In particular, the "negative symptoms" of schizophrenia, which include poor social skills, anhedonia, and apathy, are not improved by neuroleptics (Angrist, Rotrosen, & Gershon, 1980). By helping clients in these areas of functioning, groups thus may play a complementary role to medications.

This paper provides a working typology of group formats that reflect current practice. We elaborate this typology, either summarizing the literature when it is extensive or providing examples of group approaches not represented well in the literature. We offer some brief observations on effectiveness, and suggest future directions for training and research.

A TYPOLOGY OF GROUP FORMATS

Current practice has moved away from traditional group therapy in two important ways: by a shift toward greater structure, as shown by the social skills training approaches of Liberman (1988), and a shift in *locus of contact* toward greater integration into real-world activities (Stein, 1988), as exemplified by the PSR approach (Dincin, 1975; Vorspan, 1988). In Table 1 we present a typology based on these two dimensions. As is true of all typologies, ours contains some arbitrary distinctions. For example, the classification of PSR as occurring within the natural environment may be open to debate. That is, clubhouses subscribing to PSR are themselves segregated from the community; nevertheless, PSR *activities* mainly occur in integrated settings of employment, recreation, and housing.

QUADRANT I: UNSTRUCTURED APPROACHES IN SHELTERED SETTINGS

Traditional Group Therapies

Description. Diverse interactional and insight-oriented group approaches have been developed, and continue to be developed (e.g.,

Table 1. A Typology of Group Formats

	Experiential	Structured
	Quadrant I:	Quadrant II:
Artifical or Sheltered Environments	Traditional group therapy	Education groups Group skills training in a treatment setting Group residences
	Quadrant III:	Quadrant IV:
Natural Environments	Psychosocial rehabilitation Self-help group and mutual aid organizations Drop-in centers	Group skills training in natural environments

Pinder, Plante, & Howe, 1988), for clients with severe mental illness. Compared to higher functioning clients, clients with severe mental illness appear to benefit from therapy groups that provide additional *support* and *structure* (Yalom, 1983). Most practitioners also agree with Yalom's (1975) group composition principle of homogeneity for ego strength and therefore place clients with severe mental illness in separate groups from those for higher functioning clients.

Evaluation. Research on traditional group therapy for this population has yielded disappointing conclusions. Controlled evaluations have found only modest improvement in functioning for clients attending office-based group therapies (Herz, Spitzer, Gibbon, Greenspan, & Reibel, 1974; Levene, Patterson, Murphey, Overbeck, & Veach, 1970; O'Brien, Hamm, Ray, Pierce, Luborsky, & Mintz, 1972). Group therapies can boost client morale and self-esteem, provide a reference group, and normalize life experiences. They are not equipped, however, to solve the complex problems of persons with severe psychiatric disabilities. In particular, the hope in the early days of deinstitutionalization that insight-oriented therapy would enable clients to find jobs, live independently, and function in society has not been substantiated (Bond & Boyer, 1988).

Group approaches that encourage intense expression of emotion have been found to be psychologically harmful to participants with fragile self-concepts in studies with college students and mixed diagnostic groups (Lieberman, Yalom, & Miles, 1973; Yalom, Bond, Bloch, Zimmerman, & Friedman, 1977). Although these studies were targeted to higher functioning participants, the findings are consistent with research on the noxious effects of emotionally charged environments on schizophrenic relapse (Vaughn, Snyder, Freeman et al., 1984).

We agree with Parloff (1986) that the "preoccupation with group psychotherapy's efficacy in the treatment of schizophrenia is misplaced and out-of-date." Traditional group therapy for persons with severe mental illness has been eclipsed by newer developments in the field. This necessitates a reframing of evaluation questions. We do not conclude that the therapeutic use of groups with this population is now outdated, or that understanding how groups function is a futile exercise. Indeed, a shortcoming of the newer movements may be a failure to appreciate the earlier contributions of group dynamics and group therapy. Evaluation of group interventions, however, is more complex than suggested by earlier research, requiring the examination of their unique role within context of comprehensive treatment programs.

QUADRANT II: STRUCTURED APPROACHES IN SHELTERED SETTINGS

Education Groups

Description. A popular type of intervention involves providing information in a classroom format. The need for such groups arises because clients are often naive about such issues as medications (Streicker, Amdur, & Dincin, 1986), sex (Berman & Rozensky, 1984; Pepper, 1988), and substance abuse (Bergman & Harris, 1985).

Evaluation. Mazzuca's (1982) meta-analysis suggests that educational approaches are generally ineffective in increasing treatment compliance among persons with chronic physical illnesses. Didactic approaches may be even more ineffective with chronic mental illness, given the frequent additional complication of disordered thinking. A controlled evaluation of a ten-week medication education group (Streicker et al., 1986) provides direct evidence. The education group used a carefully-defined curriculum, a sensitive and motivated psychiatrist as a group leader, and peer role models. At follow-up, despite the fact that group attendance led to significant increase in knowledge and positive attitudes about drugs, clients attending the group had significantly more instances of discontinuing medications than controls. Being informed about medications was not enough to increase compliance. In fact, it may have decreased it.

Social Skills Training

Description. Group skills training is a popular group modality in mental health centers. Liberman (1988) has noted several advantages to learning social skills in a group. Groups provide naturalistic opportunities for trying out skills, an arena for ongoing assessment, and reinforcement of learned skills through peer feedback, modeling, and peer pressure to conform to positive group expectations.

Skills training, which derives from the behavioral and cognitive-behavioral traditions in psychology, starts from a premise that appears to be especially applicable to this population: Change in a particular life domain depends on interventions designed specifically for that domain (Anthony, Cohen, & Cohen, 1984).

Evaluation. Two issues are involved in evaluating the group skills-training literature: (a) Is skills training an effective technology? (b) Are groups the most efficient format to deliver this training? On the first issue, well over 50 studies have successfully implemented skills training with psychiatric patients, primarily in the area of social skills (Anthony et al., 1984; Liberman, 1988). Within a specific treatment setting, clients can be trained to perform specific interpersonal behaviors, such as: greeting, maintaining eye contact, and interviewing for a job. The research is less clear about the generalizability of these behaviors to the natural environment (Liberman, 1988). Nor has skills training yet been proven practical for training clients in a complex set of skills, such as required for maintaining employment (Bond & Boyer, 1988).

On the second issue, the group format for skills training has several practical limitations. One is the redundancy inherent in offering specific curricula to a group of clients regardless of previous attendance or individual need. Logistically it proves difficult to match clients up to appropriate groups, and most programs recycle long-term clients through groups they may not need. A second limitation is a shortage of trained staff. Given the general principle that a group leader who does not possess a particular skill cannot train clients in that skill (Anthony, 1980), trained staff are essential in this approach.

Group Residential Approaches

Description. Halfway houses have been offered as both a way to solve the housing problems caused by deinstitutionalization and a rehabilitation method. For example, Fairweather, Sanders, Maynard, Cressler, and Bleck (1969) developed a separate society, where clients could learn community living skills and work together in a small cohesive group. Other representative rehabilitation examples include Mosher (in press), Paul and Lentz (1977), and Velasquez and McCubbin (1980).

Evaluation. The above-cited studies have found reduced hospital use and higher levels of skill functioning for clients living in structured group living arrangements. However, Carling, Randolph, Blanch, and Ridgway (1988) have identified several basic flaws in group rehabilitation approaches. First, congregate living is unnatural. A recent survey has shown that such living arrangements are not most clients' first choice (Blanch, Carling, & Ridgway, 1988). Second, most group homes are transitional in nature. Clients have difficulty readjusting to new environments. When they leave the security of the group home, they suffer a reduction of supports at precisely the time they need *more*. Perhaps as a consequence, client improvement in a group residential setting often does not transfer to a new environment (Fairweather et al., 1969). Finally, congregate living may be psychologically *harmful* for clients with schizophrenia. Linn, Klett, and Caffey (1980) found that persons with schizophrenia were more likely to decompensate if placed in a foster home with three or more clients than if they were placed individually or in pairs. One possible explanation of these results is that persons with schizophrenia are vulnerable to relapse if they live in psychologically overstimulating environments (Vaughn et al., 1984).

QUADRANT III: EXPERIENTIAL IN VIVO FORMATS

Psychosocial Rehabilitation Centers

Description. Psychosocial rehabilitation (PSR) is a philosophy of rehabilitation that assumes persons with severe mental illness have "normal" needs. Group activities form the backbone of PSR programs. PSR emphasizes normalized settings, experiential learning, high expectancies for client achievement, and flexible staffing patterns (Bond, 1987; Dincin, 1975; Vorspan, 1988). PSR emphasizes pragmatic goals such as employment, independent living, and satisfying use of leisure time. Members (as clients in such programs are called) participate in a comprehensive program, with vocational, recreational, and residential components. Members are involved in PSR program governance and are made to feel *needed* for the program's success (Lanoil, 1982).

Evaluation. Several controlled and uncontrolled studies have shown that psychosocial rehabilitation programs have a positive impact on client outcomes (Beard, Pitt, Fisher, & Goertzel, 1963; Bond, Dincin, Witheridge, & Setze, 1984; Dincin & Witheridge, 1982; Malamud & McCrory, 1988). However, few studies have evaluated the efficacy of specific program components within these programs.

Farrell's (1982) work exemplifies the latter kind of evaluation. Her study of a camping program for PSR members is also unusual in its examination of the role of recreation in the rehabilitation process. Therapeutic factors in camping include the communal living experience, the novel and less complex environment suited to clients who have difficulty with ambiguity and overstimulation, and the opportunity to experience mastery through camp activities. For clients who have difficulty having fun, camping is a rare opportunity. Farrell (1982) found that members participating in a three-day camping trip showed short-term improvement in self-esteem and reduction of depression. The members' "group high" was not sustained over the long-term. However, the group cohesion they experienced appeared to contribute to their sustained attendance in PSR.

Drop-In Centers

Description. Webb (1973) has described the "therapeutic social club," which offers fellowship, recreation, and snacks within an accepting social environment. The main assumptions in this approach are that nonverbal activities encourage social activity and that open membership provides anonymity and safety for clients who avoid intimacy (Warren, 1987). Now usually referred to as "drop-in centers," these readily accessible, low-expectation programs have been used as a way to reach clients living on the fringes of society. The Los Angeles Men's Place (LAMP), located in a skid row section of that city, is one example. LAMP attracts homeless persons with major psychotic disorders. Thresholds' Lakeview Club in Chicago is designed for clients who are not suited for Thresholds' vocationally-oriented PSR program. Drop-in centers are not a recent innovation: their historical debt to social work tradition is obvious.

Evaluation. To our knowledge, there have been no rigorous evaluations of drop-in centers with this population. However, Bond, Witheridge, Wasmer, Dincin, Webb, and De Graaf-Kaser (1988), in a study of frequently hospitalized clients, used a drop-in center as a control condition. They found that less than 10% of the clients invited to the drop-in center ever attended after their initial contact. This study highlights a major drawback of drop-in centers—that members are highly self-selected. Specifically, the neediest, most isolated clients are also least likely to attend. Another selection bias has been found in urban drop-in centers: men appear much more likely to affiliate, even when some activities are specifically tailored to women.

By addressing social needs, drop-in centers may play a *complementary* role to assertive outreach programs. Case workers who make home visits are effective in addressing practical needs, but their clients continue to report feelings of loneliness and dissatisfaction with structuring free time (Bond et al., 1988b). Thus a natural development is for a home-visiting program to add a drop-in center component to their services (Bond, Miller, Krumwied, & Ward, 1988).

Self-Help Groups and Mutual Aid Societies

Description. In 1982 Estroff prophetically suggested self-help as the "next step" for consumers of mental health services. Indeed, many new self-help organizations have formed and expanded in the past two decades. NIMH recently has begun nurturing consumer groups. There are many types, ranging from "partnership" to "separatist" groups (Stroul, 1986). Some traditional groups, such as Recovery and GROW, emphasize mutual support (Kurtz & Chambon, 1987). Others have a more political action and advocacy component (Chamberlin, Roger, & Sneed, 1989). The National Mental Health Consumers' Association is an umbrella organization for groups representing more of the activist and advocacy side of the spectrum. Another variation, now found in projects in Michigan, Colorado, and Philadelphia, is the use of consumer volunteers to assist other consumers—in essence, developing a new cadre of case managers (Mowbray, Wellwood, & Chamberlin, 1988).

Evaluation. Research on the efficacy of mental health self-help groups is virtually nonexistent. However, their popularity has spawned speculations about how they help members. A widely-held theory is that self-help groups provide members an ideology for combating self-defeating attitudes (Antze, 1979). Another hypothesis is the "helper-therapy principle" (Riessman, 1965), which states that helpers (e.g., consumer-volunteers) receive benefit in the process of reaching out to others. Otteson (1979) successfully applied the helper-therapy principle in a psychiatric hospital. He showed that inpatients benefited more from a "buddy system" than a self-oriented therapy. Finally, one obvious role for self-help groups is providing long-term social support that is sorely lacking in many clients' lives.

Many of the strengths and weaknesses of drop-in centers also apply to self-help groups. In both cases self-selection is evident. In contrast to drop-in centers, women are more likely to join mutual aid groups (Young & Williams, 1988). Moreover, some surveys suggest that the large majority of active members in traditional mutual aid organizations would not meet the criteria for chronic mental illness (Antze, 1979; Rappaport, 1988; Young & Williams, 1988). Although not ruling out the potential for these groups to provide an "ecological niche" for clients who otherwise would not fit into the mental health system (Rappaport, 1988; Salem, Seidman, & Rappaport, 1988), we do not foresee these groups filling a void for the "revolving door" clients, as Rappaport has hypothesized.

QUADRANT IV: STRUCTURED IN VIVO FORMATS

Clear examples of structured group approaches that are truly within the natural environment are difficult to find. One possible example may be some group variants of the "supported employment" (SE) model. SE is an attempt to train clients after placing them in competitive employment sites (Bond, 1987). Even so, when a group of clients is placed together in an employment site, the resulting enclave may resemble a segregated work environment. Another possible example is "supported training." In Boston University's Continuing Education Program young adults with psychiatric disabilities take courses together at the university and receive guidance from a graduate student with whom each is paired (Unger,

Danley, Kohn, & Hutchinson, 1987). Evaluations of supported employment and training are just beginning to emerge in the literature, and an assessment of these is premature.

DISCUSSION

Directions for Training

University training has fallen short in providing persons working in public mental health with needed skills. Although providing appropriate training in generic counseling skills, universities have not provided adequate training for work with the psychiatric population. With some noteworthy exceptions, PSR and CSP concepts have not been well-integrated into the curricula of schools of social work (Davis, in press). Another area for consciousness-raising might be the role of self-help groups as a major mental health resource (Kurtz, Mann, & Chambon, 1988).

Whether the training is done at the preservice or inservice level, trainees need to be exposed to positive models of effective programs. NIMH has recently encouraged collaboration between universities and public mental health to foster relevant academic training.

Directions for Research

Group norms. An underlying assumption of PSR is that members change by their exposure to the norms and culture of the PSR clubhouse, in which they are accepted and needed (Lanoil, 1982). Although intuitively appealing, this theory has never been systematically tested. Similarly, self-help groups provide a profound shift in perspective in viewing one's illness that is presumed to be therapeutic. Preliminary work in a PSR setting (Ryan, Bell, & Metcalf, 1982), group residences (Mosher, in press), self-help groups (Rappaport, 1988), and outpatient therapy groups (Bond, 1983) demonstrate that group norms can be studied.

Group leadership. The extensive research literature on leadership factors in group therapy (Dies, 1983) has been virtually ignored in programs serving persons with severe mental illness. The PSR model has made peer leadership an article of faith. PSR assumes a strong action orientation, in which staff work side-by-side with clients, rather than maintaining a professional distance (Dincin, 1975; Lanoil, 1982). These assumptions should be tested empirically. Mosher (in press) noted the following self-selection factors for residential staff: prior experience coping with significant life stresses, a practical problem-solving orientation, and nonauthoritarian attitudes.

Dropouts. In the older group therapy literature, dropouts were a familiar concern (Bond & Lieberman, 1978). Recommendations for reducing dropouts included "role preparation" for lower-class, "psychologically unsophisticated" clients to inoculate them from the stresses of early therapy sessions (e.g., Heitler, 1973). It now appears that assertive outreach is necessary to engage some clients in treatment (Bond et al., 1988a; 1988b).

Negative effects of groups. The advantages of placing clients in homogeneous groups must be weighed against their potential negative impact. For example, the issue of "institutional dependency" (Bond & Boyer, 1988) must always be considered whenever clients are trained together in a sheltered environment. Perhaps a way to clarify the positive and negative normative effects of groups would be to compare clients attending a PSR program to those receiving assertive community treatment (Stein & Test, 1980), an approach that uses individualized treatment within the natural environment.

CONCLUSION

Group therapy as a microcosm of the real world in which clients learn new behavioral patterns (Yalom, 1975) has limitations as a model for clients with severe mental illness. Group therapy has been modified to make the learning more concrete. The two ways for doing this are: (a) train clients in a real environment, not a simulated one; and (b) train clients specifically in skills they will need, rather than providing general support and hoping they make the translation. Research and academic training has lagged behind current practice. An extensive research literature on group dynamics and group leadership is a starting point for building an empirically-based framework for groups for persons with severe mental illness.

REFERENCES

Angrist, B. J., Rotrosen, J., & Gershon, S. (1980). Positive and negative symptoms in schizophrenia—Differential response to amphetamine and neuroleptics. *Psychopharmacology*, *72*, 17-19.

Anthony, W. A. (1980). *The principles of psychiatric rehabilitation*. Baltimore· University Park Press.

Anthony, W. A., Cohen, M. R., & Cohen, B. F. (1984). Psychiatric rehabilitation. In J. A. Talbott (Ed.), *The chronic mental patient Five years later* (pp. 137-157). Orlando, Florida Grune & Stratton.

Antze, P. (1979). Role of ideologies in peer psychotherapy groups. In M. A. Lieberman & L. D. Borman (Eds.), *Self-help groups for coping with crisis* (pp. 272-304) San Francisco Jossey-Bass.

Beard, J. H., Pitt, R. B., Fisher, S. H., & Goertzel, V. (1963). Evaluating the effectiveness of a psychiatric rehabilitation program. *American Journal of Orthopsychiatry*, *33*, 701-712.

Berman, C., & Rozensky, R. H. (1984). Sex education for the chronic psychiatric patient· The effects of a sexual-issues group on knowledge and attitudes *Psychosocial Rehabilitation Journal*, *8* (1), 28-34.

Bergman, H. C., & Harris, M. (1985). Substance abuse among young adult chronic patients. *Psychosocial Rehabilitation Journal*, *9* (1), 49-54.

Blanch, A. K., Carling, P. J., & Ridgway, P (1988) Normal housing with specialized supports· A psychiatric rehabilitation approach to living in the community. *Rehabilitation Psychology*, *33*, 47-55.

Bond, G. R. (1983). Norm regulation in therapy groups In R R. Dies & K R. MacKenzie (Eds.), *Advances in group psychotherapy* (pp. 171-189) New York International Universities Press.

Bond, G. R. (1987). Supported work as a modification of the transitional employment model for clients with psychiatric disabilities. *Psychosocial Rehabilitation Journal*, *11*(2), 55-75.

Bond, G. R., & Boyer, S. L. (1988). Rehabilitation programs and outcomes. In J. A. Ciardiello & M. D. Bell (Eds.), *Vocational rehabilitation of persons with prolonged mental illness* (pp. 231-263). Baltimore, MD Johns Hopkins Press.

Bond, G. R., Dincin, J., Setze, P. J , & Witheridge, T. F (1984) The effectiveness of psychiatric rehabilitation A summary of research at Thresholds *Psychosocial Rehabilitation Journal*, 7(4), 6-22

Bond, G. R , & Lieberman, M. A (1978). Selection criteria for group therapy In K. Brodie & P. Brady (Eds.), *Controversy in psychiatry* (pp. 679-702). Philadelphia W. B Saunders Co.

Bond, G R , Miller, L. D , Krumwied, R. D., & Ward, R S (1988a) Assertive case management in three CMHCs A controlled study. *Hospital and Community Psychiatry*, *39*, 411-418.

Bond, G. R., Witheridge, T. F., Dincin, J , Wasmer, D., Webb, J., De Graaf-Kaser, R. (1988b) *Assertive outreach and service coordination for frequent users of psychiatric hospitals in a large city: A controlled study* Unpublished manuscript.

Carling, P. J , Randolph, F. L., Blanch, A. K., & Ridgway, P. (1988). A review of the research on housing and community integration for people with psychiatric disabilities. *NARIC Quarterly, 1* (3), 1, 6-18.

Chamberlin, J , Rogers, J. A., & Sneed, C. S. (1989). Consumers, families, and community support systems. *Psychosocial Rehabilitation Journal, 12* (3), 92-106

Davis, K. E. (Ed.) (in press). *Social work research and utilization: Strengthening science-based education for services to the long-term seriously mentally ill.* Proceedings from a forum presented by the National Association of Deans and Directors of Schools of Social Work, September 29-30, 1988, Arlington, VA.

Dies, R. R. (1983). Clinical implications of research on leadership in short-term group psychotherapy. In R. R. Dies and K. R. MacKenzie (Eds.), *Advances in group psychotherapy· Integrating research and practice* (pp. 27-78). New York· International Universities Press

Dincin, J. (1975). Psychiatric rehabilitation. *Schizophrenia Bulletin, 1*, 131-148.

Dincin, J., & Witheridge, T. F. (1982). Psychiatric rehabilitation as a deterrent to recidivism. *Hospital and Community Psychiatry, 33*, 645-650.

Estroff, S. E. (1982). The next step. Self-help. *Hospital and Community Psychiatry, 33*, 609.

Fairweather, G. W., Sanders, D. H., Maynard, H., Cressler, D. L., & Bleck, D S. (1969). *Community life for the mentally ill.* Chicago Aldine.

Farrell, D. M. (1982) *Effects of a wilderness camping experience on emotionally disturbed adolescents' self-esteem, closeness, and symptomatology*. Unpublished master's thesis, Southern Illinois University.

Goldman, H. H., Gattozzi, A. A., & Taube, C. A. (1981). Defining and counting the chronically mentally ill. *Hospital and Community Psychiatry, 32*, 21-27.

Heitler, J. B. (1973). Preparation of lower-class patients for expressive group psychotherapy. *Journal of Consulting and Clinical Psychology, 41*, 251-260.

Herz, M. I., Spitzer, R. L., Gibbon, M., Greenspan, K., & Reibel, S. (1974). Individual versus group aftercare treatment. *American Journal of Psychiatry, 131*, 808-812.

Kanas, N. (1986). Group therapy with schizophrenics· A review of controlled studies. *International Journal of Group Psychotherapy, 36*, 339-351.

Kurtz, L. F., & Chambon, A. (1987). Comparison of self-help groups for mental health *Health and Social Work, 12*, 275-283.

Kurtz, L. F., Mann, K. B., & Chambon, A. (1988). Linking between social workers and mental health mutual-aid groups. *Social Work in Health Care, 13*, 69-78.

Lanoil, J. (1982). An analysis of the psychiatric psychosocial rehabilitation center. *Psychosocial Rehabilitation Journal, 5*(1), 55-59.

Levene, H. L., Patterson, V., Murphey, B. G., Overbeck, A. L., & Veach, T. L. (1970). The aftercare of schizophrenics An evaluation of group and individual approaches *Psychiatric Quarterly, 44*, 296-304.

Liberman, R. P. (1988). *Psychiatric rehabilitation of chronic mental patients*. Washington, DC: American Psychiatric Association Press.

Lieberman, M. A., Yalom, I. D., & Miles, M. B. (1973). *Encounter groups: First facts*. New York: Basic Books.

Linn, M. W., Klett, J., Caffey, E. M. (1980). Foster home characteristics and psychiatric patient outcome: The wisdom of Gheel confirmed. *Archives of General Psychiatry*, *37*, 129-132.

Luborsky, L., Singer, R., & Luborsky, L. (1975). Comparative studies of psychotherapies. *Archives of General Psychiatry*, *32*, 995-1008.

Malamud, T. J., & McCrory, D. J. (1988). Transitional employment and psychosocial rehabilitation. In J. A. Ciardiello and M. D. Bell (Eds.), *Vocational rehabilitation for persons with prolonged mental illness* (pp. 150-162). Baltimore, MD: Johns Hopkins Press.

Mazzuca, S. A. (1982). Does patient education in chronic disease have therapeutic value? *Journal of Chronic Disease*, *35*, 521-529.

Mosher, L. R. (in press). Community residential treatment/alternatives to hospitalization. In A. Bellack (Ed.), *A clinical guide for the treatment of schizophrenia*. New York: Plenum Press.

Mosher, L. R., & Keith, S. J. (1980). Psychosocial treatment: Individual, group, family, and community support approaches. *Schizophrenia Bulletin*, *1*, 10-41.

Mowbray, C. T., Wellwood, R., Chamberlain, P. (1988). Project Stay: A consumer-run support service. *Psychosocial Rehabilitation Journal*, *12* (1), 33-42.

O'Brien, C. P., Hamm, K. B., Ray, B. A., Pierce, J. F., Luborsky, L., & Mintz, J. (1972). Group versus individual psychotherapy with schizophrenics: A controlled outcome study. *Archives of General Psychiatry*, *27*, 474-478.

Otteson, J. P. (1979). Curative caring: The use of buddy groups with chronic schizophrenics. *Journal of Consulting and Clinical Psychology*, *47*, 649-651.

Parloff, M. B. (1986). Discussion of "Group therapy with schizophrenics." *International Journal of Group Psychotherapy*, *36*, 353-360.

Paul, G. L., & Lentz, R. J. (1977). *Psychosocial treatment of the chronic mental patient*. Cambridge: Harvard University Press.

Pepper, E. (1988). Sexual awareness groups in a psychiatric day treatment program. *Psychosocial Rehabilitation Journal*, *11* (3), 45-52.

Pinder, S. L., Plante, T. G., & Howe, D. (1988, August). *Introducing the Living with Illness Group: Specialized treatment of patients with chronic schizophrenic conditions*. Presentation at the annual convention of the American Psychological Association, Atlanta, GA.

Rappaport, J. (1988, August). *GROW, A mutual-aid society*. Presentation given at the Region V Community Support Conference, Chicago, IL.

Riessman, F. (1965). The "helper-therapy" principle. *Social Work*, *10*, 27-32.

Ryan, E. P., Bell, M. D., & Metcalf, J. C. (1982). The development of a rehabilitation psychology program for persons with schizophrenia: Changes in the treatment environment. *Rehabilitation Psychology*, *27*, 67-85.

Salem, D. A., Seidman, E., Rappaport, J. (1988). Community treatment of the

mentally ill: The promise of mutual-help organizations. *Social Work, 33*, 403-408.
Scott, D., & Griffith, M. (1982). The evaluation of group therapy in the treatment of schizophrenia. *Small Group Behavior, 13*, 415-422.
Stein, L. I. (1988). "It's the focus, not the locus." Hocus-Pocus! *Hospital and Community Psychiatry, 39*, 1029.
Stein, L. I., & Test, M. A. (1980). An alternative to mental health treatment. I: Conceptual model, treatment program, and clinical evaluation. *Archives of General Psychiatry, 37*, 392-397.
Streicker, S. K., Amdur, M., & Dincin, J. (1986). Educating patients about psychiatric medications: Failure to enhance compliance. *Psychosocial Rehabilitation Journal, 9* (4), 15-28.
Stroul, B. A. (1986). *Models of community support services: Approaches to helping persons with long-term mental illness*. Boston: Center for Psychiatric Rehabilitation.
Stroul, B. A. (1989). Introduction to the Special Issue The Community Support System Concept. *Psychosocial Rehabilitation Journal, 12* (3), 5-8.
Turner, J. C., & TenHoor, W. J. (1978). The NIMH Community Support Program Pilot approach to a needed social reform. *Schizophrenia Bulletin, 4*, 319-348.
Unger, K. V., Danley, K. S., Kohn, L., & Hutchinson, D. (1987) Rehabilitation through education A university-based continuing education program for young adults with psychiatric disabilities on a university campus. *Psychosocial Rehabilitation Journal, 10* (3), 35-49.
Vaughn, C. E., Snyder, K. S., Freeman, W. et al. (1984). Family factors in schizophrenic relapse. *Archives of General Psychiatry, 41*, 1169-1177.
Velasquez, J. S., & McCubbin, H. I. (1980). Towards establishing the effectiveness of community-based residential treatment Program evaluation by experimental research. *Journal of Social Service Research, 3*, 337-359.
Vorspan, R. (1988). Activities of daily living in the clubhouse You can't vacuum in a vacuum. *Psychosocial Rehabilitation Journal, 12*(2), 15-21.
Warren, P. The therapeutic social club: A collectivity for ex-psychiatric patients. *Social Work with Groups, 9* (4), 91-101.
Webb, L. J (1973). The therapeutic social club. American *Journal of Occupational Therapy, 27*, 81-83.
Yalom, I. D. (1975). *The theory and practice of group psychotherapy*. New York Basic Books.
Yalom, I. D. (1983). *Inpatient group psychotherapy*. New York: Basic Books.
Yalom, I. D., Bond, G. R., Bloch, S. T., Zimmerman, E., & Friedman, L. (1977). The impact of a weekend group experience on individual therapy. *Archives of General Psychiatry, 34*, 399-415.
Young, J., & Williams, C L. (1988). Whom do mutual-help groups help? A typology of members. *Hospital and Community Psychiatry, 39*, 1178-1182.

Group Exposure: A Method of Treating Agoraphobia

Sheldon D. Rose

SUMMARY. Group exposure method is a broad based procedure used primarily in the treatment of agoraphobia and social phobias. It is a strategy with extensive empirical support for its efficacy. This research is reviewed in the article. The primary approach of the program is to help client confront in the real world the specific situations that clients complain they are unable to endure. The group is used to provide the clients with mutual support in the process of confrontation. Meetings involve preparing for excursions into the real world, the confrontation itself, and finally back to the meeting room for an evaluation of the experience and mutual reinforcment for success. Like other methods in this approach, the specific activities of clients and group worker vary from phase to phase in treatment. If the group is to succeed attention must also be paid to the group variables which either impede or enhance the progress of treatment. The procedure may be the major intervention strategy or may be used in combination with a variety of other procedures for attaining and maintaining the remediation of agoraphobia and other complaints the client brings to the treatment situation. For those group workers who work with clients with inordinate fears especially, agoraphobia, this is a method, by virtue of its empirical support, meriting extensive consideration.

Client in group of agoraphobics: I don't go anywhere any more. I couldn't have even come today if my mother hadn't come with me. Even that didn't shake my fear that something awful would happen. It seems it just started a few years ago when I was twenty, and it's been getting worse all the time. I

Sheldon D. Rose is affiliated with the School of Social Work, University of Wisconsin, Madison, WI.

> try. I really do! But as soon as I go out I have these terrible anxiety attacks. I feel like I'm going to die. Maybe it would be better I'm just a useless human being. I'm so alone.

Agoraphobia, literally, fear of the market place, has been described in the literature since the time of the ancient Greeks (Marks, 1969). More currently defined as fear of public places, or fear of fear, agoraphobia is commonly discovered by therapists in various treatment contexts. In addition to an intense fear of leaving the home and going into public places, most agoraphobics suffer from fear of fear, lack of assertion, debilitating panic, low level of self sufficiency and high levels of "free floating anxiety" (Goldstein & Chambliss, 1978). Not uncommon, too, are complaints of depression and depersonalization. The panic attacks are characterized by a rapidly pounding heart, inability to breathe, and faintness. These symptoms are often interpreted by the clients as sign of impending death or going "crazy" (Marks, 1970). Marks also notes that once begun, these problems tend to fluctuate over the span of a lifetime. The most common models of treatment have been the psychoanalytic (Stamm, 1972) and the medical model (Zitrin, Klein, Lindemann, Tobak, Rock, Kaplan & Ganz, 1976). More recently various social learning models (e.g., Wolpe, 1973, and Marks, 1970) have evolved. One of these social learning approaches lends itself in particular to group treatment, the group exposure method.

The group exposure method, first reported on as group approach by Watson, Mullet and Pillay (1973) and Hand, LaMontagne and Marks (1974), is an in vivo procedure in which the agoraphobic client is treated in groups by means of confrontation in the real world with or prolonged exposure to the objects of their fear. The clients not only discuss with the others going into various public places such as the streets, markets, and crowded buses, but they actually draw up a plan together and then carry it out as a group.

The group exposure method should be of particular interest to group workers using a goal oriented paradigm because of its well developed set of treatment parameters. It readily lends itself to a multimethod approach since it draws upon cognitive restructuring, relaxation, the modeling sequence, self reinforcement and many other behavioral procedures discussed in detail elsewhere (e.g., see

Rose & Edleson, 1987). However group exposure has some unique characteristics which are discussed in this article which differentiate it from other behavioral strategies. Group exposure has a number of advantages over other treatment procedures used in the treatment of agoraphobia. It is one of the few approaches to the treatment of agoraphobia that has empirical support (some of which is discussed below). In addition, as Hand et al. (1974) point out problem-focussed retraining under real-life conditions (reality testing) as group-therapeutic fieldwork can be a means of treatment in its own right, it may open up the patient for subsequent attempts to tackle more complex problems, or it may just be an adjunct in a multilevel approach such as the one outlined in this book. Another important characteristic may be that it may prevent drop-outs from treatment. In a study by Haffner and Marks (1976) in which group and individual exposure approaches were compared, all drop-outs were from the individual condition. Another advantage is that group exposure has applications in the treatment of other anxiety related disorders such as social phobia. Finally repeated studies have shown that the group is at least as effective as individual exposure but more efficient (Haffner & Marks, 1976).

Most of the other empirical support for group exposure treatment of agoraphobia is derived from the work of Hand et al. (1974), Watson et al. (1973), Teasdale, Walsh, Lancashire and Mathews (1977), Haffner and Marks, (1976), and Telch, Agras, Taylor, Barr, Roth, Walton and Gallen (1985). In none of these studies were treatment control groups used, but patients in each of the studies showed significant before-after changes in terms of their ability to approach the phobic object. In the study by Telch et al. (1985) the changes were significantly enhanced by a combination of pharmacological agents and group exposure, although in most studies on pharmacological agents, the results have been mixed. Emmelkamp and Mersch, 1982, showed that group exposure was superior to cognitive restructuring on the in-vivo test but on that same test there were no significant differences at follow up.

The purpose of this article is to acquaint the group worker with the potential of the group exposure method to the treatment of agoraphobia and other phobic disorders. In order to establish the differentiated role of the clinician in the application of group exposure across time, the role is first described as it applied in the various phases of treatment.

PHASES OF TREATMENT

As in most behavioral and cognitive behavioral approaches the treatment process can be broken down into a number of overlapping phases of worker activity. These include orientation, assessment, cohesion-building, intervention, resolution of group problems, generalization training and termination. Let us examine each of these phases in terms of the activity of the group worker and the typical client responses for each phase.

Orientation

As in most procedures the clients are first presented with a theoretical justification and a description of what they can expect. This occurs initially in the pre-group interview. The orientation message is repeated at the first session in order to make sure that everyone understands what is about to happen. (For an excellent example, see Emmelkamp, 1982.) Generally, clients are assured that they will not be forced to do anything they do not want to do or feel will bring about panic. This assurance is essential not only for sound ethical reasons, but also to prevent the clients from immediately dropping out of treatment. The reasons for being in the group are also explained (e.g., mutual support, sharing experiences, seeing that one is not alone with this very serious problem, and learning an effective strategy for dealing with their problem). Considerable attention is invested in a behavioral explanation of phobic behavior, on the irrational elements attached to it, and how the group will be structured. Stressed in this presentation is the fact that feared situations will be presented in such a way as to gradually help them to face the day to day events that shape their world. In the orientation sessions a great deal of time is permitted for questions and reassurance that the clients will not be forced to do anything they do not want to do.

Assessment and Goal Setting

In general clients come (or more commonly are brought) to agencies or a private practitioner with many anxiety related problems. Among these problems are fear of going out in the world or intense fear of coming in contact with other people. The scope and incapacitating problems are usually determined by the worker in an interview. On the basis of the interview a decision is made whether to include the client in the group, to refer elsewhere, or to obtain additional information. For those included in the group they are usually asked to monitor their own approach behavior. A self-monitoring checklist seems to be the most effective means of continuing assessment of approach behaviors to the phobic objects and a determination of anxiety levels. During the follow-up period the client is asked to mail the form monthly to the group leader. Some workers also use an idiosyncratically developed Behavioral Avoidance scale (B.A.T.) (Jansson, Jeremalm & Ost, 1984) which is a hierarchy of approximately 15 agoraphobic situations determined in the intake situation. The client attempts to complete as many of these environmental encounters as possible before and after treatment and at follow-up. When the form is received, the client receives a telephone call to discuss setbacks and difficulties encountered.

While assessment is taking place, the group worker begins to take steps to enhance the cohesion of the group. The strategies used are discussed briefly in the following section.

Cohesion-Building Phase

As in all group methods if the group is to be effective, a focus on building the cohesion of the group is essential. Groups characterized by cooperation, mutual interpersonal liking, attraction to the leader, concern for each other are far more powerful group reinforcers for trying out the potentially panic inducing behaviors than groups in which these characteristics are absent. In the treatment of agoraphobia, Hand et al. (1974) found that subjects in high cohesive groups had a lower drop-out rate than those in the low cohesive groups although the outcomes of those who remained were comparable. As a result of the importance of cohesion in order to encourage its growth such strategies are employed as the use of food at sessions, the use of intra-group exercises which support high participation by all members, the use of role playing, the maximum involvement of all members at all meetings, the avoidance of excessive pressure, the use of large amount of positive reinforcement and group support for all accomplishments, and the use of variation in programming. These are the same procedures used in other types of groups but failure to address the issue of cohesion planfully often result in the lowering of the effectiveness of that group.

Intervention Phase

Interventions consist of (1) preparation for exposure; (2) group exposure; (3) evaluation of the exposure experience and (4) homework in which exposure is carried out by the client as an extra-group assignment. During the preparation clients are trained in anxiety management procedures by means of worker and member modeling, simulated practice, and group discussion of any spontaneous accomplishments that occurred since the last session. In addition the group members discuss the homework they have completed during the week. The major focus in the preparation part of the meeting is on the particular exposure exercise they will be performing at the given session. Often after a discussion of the exercise, the members will cognitively rehearse step by step what they will be doing shortly in the real world. In the extra-group exposure period, the group members leave the meeting room and go out in the real world together to face the anxiety producing situations.

There are a number of variations in the actual exposure of the clients to public places. One most commonly used variation is that described by Emmelkamp and Kuipers (1985). The group goes out together and members support each other in the process. They are encouraged not to hold on to each other but are permitted to walk, at first near each other. After a given period of time, the members are encouraged to walk at some distance from each other. Finally each goes off a little way on their own. The group then returns together to the place where the group was meeting originally (either the same day or more often at the following session) to discuss their experiences during the exposure period and then develop homework for themselves to perform similar activities on their own between sessions. In general the homework assumed by each client should not go beyond the level of difficulty practiced in the session. If possible some form of monitoring of the homework assignment is advised. Homework is always reviewed at the beginning of the next session.

Generally, a graduated program (from activities that are mildly anxiety producing to those that are highly anxiety producing) is used initially so as not to provoke an anxiety attack. Examples of high anxiety producing events commonly used are shopping in a crowded supermarket, riding in a filled elevator, taking a crowded bus. The group together can be used to determine a hierarchy of events leading to the most fear inducing ones.

The speed with which individuals are able to carry out the graduated exposure exercises varies from person to person. Rather than creating a problem, the clients who progress more rapidly can be encouraged to serve as a model for those who progress less rapidly. Moreover clients are assured that each is permitted to function at his or her own individualized speed in order to avoid a panic attack. Nevertheless, it sometimes happens that the slower clients express jealousy of the progress of the more rapidly achieving clients. Following the suggestion of Emmelkamp and Kuipers (1985) group workers are urged to constantly point out that such differences will exist throughout treatment and that it works against individuals to compare themselves with others. This concern, should it arise, can also be dealt with as a group problem.

Gustavson, Jansson, Jerremalm and Ost (1985), who systematically examined worker behaviors during individual exposure sessions, found that the most frequent practitioner behaviors during intervention were praise, empathy, and feedback while "challenge, reminders of negative consequences, and explicit demands" were least often used. The implication is that exposure is basically a positive approach rather than a confrontative one. In groups one could expect the same behaviors on the part of the group worker and encouragement by the group worker of the same behaviors on the part of the members to each other.

Group Problem Resolution

This phase can actually occur at any time in the history of the group, although it is most likely to occur after the intervention phase begins. The threat of actually having to face the feared event in the natural environment will often trigger off such group problems as interpersonal comparisons (mentioned above), lowering of cohesion, mutual disagreement with all plans, a common criticism of the worker, a common failure to do homework, absenteeism, pairing off in the group meetings, disruptive behavior in the group meeting. Usually a statement of what the group worker feels is happening, plus encouragement to move on with the program is sufficient to handle the problem. Initial successes seem to resolve these group problems. If not, a halting of the formal agenda and a discussion of what the group worker perceives to be happening in the group. If the members experience the situation as a problem, it will be followed by systematic problem solving which provides an opportunity for the group to resolve the problem. In our experience failure to deal with the emerging group problem often results in failure of the group to meet the goals of the clients.

Generalization Phase

The purpose of most treatment, regardless of its orientation, is not only to achieve change but to transfer what has been learned in the clinical setting to the real world and to maintain that what has been learned long after treatment has terminated. The fact that the behavior is actually performed in the real world with real world problems reduces the distance required to transfer change. The fact that most of the group session actually occurs in the real world is a unique characteristic of the exposure approach. With most methods this is not possible. In group exposure, only the in-group activities need eventually to be faded.

An important principle of maintaining change is preparation for set-backs. Mathews, Gelder and Johnston (1981) made use of an individualized set-back list for each patient. Such a list contained instructions as to what to do in case of a set-back. The principles outlined were to go back to the anxiety producing situation as soon as possible, to take one step back in practice and rehearse that step often, to brush up the coping instructions, and to remind oneself of previous gains. In addition, Jansson et al. (1984) warned patients about high risk situations such as holidays, sickness, conflicts at work and with spouses and they were prepared to make use of the set-back strategies in those situations. Jansson et al. (1984) found that patients receiving this preparation for set-backs improved on 34% of the items on the BAT at pre-test, 76% at post tests and that same percentage was maintained at the six month follow up.

Another procedure used in maintaining gains obtained in the group treatment of agoraphobics was the use of self-help groups (Sinnott, Jones, Scott-Fordham & Woodward, 1982). Although increasing the dependence of some external source of support, the self-help group reduces the dependency on the group worker and other professional staff.

Another way of fading the dependence on the group is to use a buddy system where the homework is done in pairs or triads before the client tries it out on his or her own. Thus, homework, too, plays a major role in the transfer of learning from the group supported practice to the actual performance, first in dyads then eventually alone, of the previous feared activity.

Another principle of generalization is that the clients be maximally involved in their own treatment. Clients who make decisions about what happens to them in treatment appear to maintain what they have done better than those who are told what to do. In the latter case as soon as the worker disappears, the change disappears also. None of the authors cited above address specifically how the clients are involved in the exposure process. It appears at first glance that it is something done to the client and from which he gets better. In practice that is rarely the case. It is our experience that the clients are involved in a number of ways. First, each person decides for him or herself the exercises or parts of exercises to be completed. Although the general form of the exercise is proposed to the group, the members are involved together in the first part of a session in the design of the exercise and their involvement in planning increases over time. They are involved in the evaluation of outcome and suggestions for new approaches that might be used. There is great deal of client-self determination.

Rather than prepare people for the trauma of termination, clients are prepared to function independently of the group. However, in order to avoid dramatic termination, booster sessions are commonly held at a one month, two month and then a six month interval.

During this period the clients are asked to self-monitor their activities in the real world. At the sessions they report their successes and failures, and plans are made how to deal with set-backs and prepare for the next booster session.

GROUP ORGANIZATIONAL PRINCIPLES

There are a number of variations in size of group, number of sessions and other organizational variables. In early studies Hand et al. (1974) and Teasdale et al. (1977) had three five-hour sessions. Some authors met as infrequently as once a week but for 11 sessions. Still others expanded this to as many as three hours sessions a week for 10 weeks (Emmelkamp & Kuipers, 1979). Foa, Turner, Jameson and Payne (1980) found that 10 three-hour sessions on a daily basis was more effective than 10 weekly sessions. One could surmise that this may have been due to the fact that groups with massed sessions were more cohesive than groups which met only weekly. Most programs however have two to three sessions a week for purely practical reasons (see, e.g., Emmelkamp & Kuipers, 1979) and most programs last from 6 to 10 sessions with the modal number about 8. Most sessions last for two to three hours. For the reasons mentioned above and for purely practical reasons, I prefer 10 sessions of three hours each.

The number of clients in each group varies from five to eight. However in the larger groups the actual exposure exercises are usually carried out in smaller subgroups of three to four people.

AN EXAMPLE OF GROUP EXPOSURE

As a result of an advertisement in the center's newsletter, seven women indicated an interest in a group for people who found it difficult if not impossible to leave their homes alone. In initial telephone contact the group worker explained the program and assured the women that they would never be forced to do anything they did not want to do. At the first meeting six showed up all of whom were accompanied by a relative or friend. After some discussion of the assumptions of the approach and the theory of agoraphobia, the group worker brought in a guest who told of her experience with the procedure. After some discussion the group agreed that it was also necessary to do something active about their problem. The group worker handed out a set of activities used in other groups which the members examined. After some discussion and evaluation the members selected a set of activities that they agreed to carry out together in small groups. These activities included shopping at a shopping mall, going to a movie together, making the rounds of a number of church singles groups in subgroups of three and four, going to other activities where other single people would be present, making a second visit and talking to three people whom they did not know, going on a two day bus tour in subgroups, going to a crowded dance with their subgroups, and finally going to any social activity alone. The members agreed to monitor weekly their participation in each of these activities and the length of time spent in the given activity. The group worker helped the members to set up a number of procedures for handling panic or intense anxiety should it occur such as deep breathing and concentration. It was important to mutually encourage each other to do what they agreed upon but not to pressure them unduly, everyone had his or her own tempo. The group worker emphasized that it was important to look only at one's own level of achievement and not others because of the difference in tempo and the severity of the problem. Following completion of the first subgroup exercise of going together to a crowded shopping center the members returned to the meeting place and reported back to the others how well it worked, analyzed any cognitive distortions such as people would see that "I'm crazy with fear," and other discussed difficulties that occurred and how they handled it. The importance of relaxation was stressed by several of the women. At the meeting there was a lot of mutual support for their achievement and they shared a sense of accomplishment. They then modified the next step somewhat by agreeing to spend some time alone, asking for help from the clerk, and asking someone for the time. These were role played in the group. They assigned these modifications as homework assignments to each other to be done in pairs or in a triad during the week. A similar pattern was carried out at the next nine sessions over a five week period.

The results of the procedure were the achievement of treatment goals of participating once a week in some social event where single people were present for four of the six people in the group. Two others were still relying on a buddy to go out to these places but could talk to people when the buddy stood at a distance. However, they noted that they had plans to take the next step the following week and used the meeting to prepare for it. One person had dropped the group following the first group exposure session. A post group telephone call revealed that she was in individual treatment and that her therapist had advised her to drop the group. No reason was given.

BEYOND GROUP EXPOSURE FOR AGORAPHOBIA

Group exposure is almost always combined with other treatment methods as in the above example. Since many of the clients who complain about agoraphobia manifest interpersonal problems other than the reason for which they originally came for treatment, we have added modeling, problem solving, and cognitive-restructuring methods to group exposure. Also utilized are coping skill training, group reinforcement methods, group discussion, and relaxation methods as a means of preparing the clients for the extra-group exposure phase. Research does not yet lend support to any particular set of preparatory procedures, but practice experience suggests the effectiveness of the above procedures. Moreover, some empirical support exists for the use of problem solving and cognitive restructuring (Kanter & Goldfried, 1979) in the treatment of agoraphobia.

Other Uses of Exposure Methods

Although group exposure methods have been applied primarily to agoraphobics, similar procedures could and probably should be applied in other areas as well. For example, Emmelkamp, Mersch, Vissia and Van Der Helm ran such a group for social phobics. They had such problems as fear of blushing, fear their hands would tremble in front of others, fear of speaking to strangers and making inquiries in shops and offices, and fear of giving speeches. The authors compared exposure in vivo in groups, with rational emotive therapy and self instructional training (n = 34). They found that the cognitive strategies worked as well as the exposure strategies on all the performance criteria. In the exposure methods the clients had to confront their feared situations in the group. For example, clients who were afraid of blushing had to sit in front of others with an open necked blouse until anxiety dissipated. Those afraid their hands would tremble had to serve tea to each member of the group. Similar assignments were carried out as a group in the town center.

CONCLUSION

Group exposure method is a broad based procedure used primarily in the treatment of agoraphobia. It is a strategy with some empirical support for its efficacy in the treatment of agoraphobia and social phobias. The primary aspects of the program are to help clients confront the specific situations that clients complain they are unable to endure. The group is used to provide the clients with mutual support in the process of confrontation. Meetings involve preparing for excursions into the real world, the confrontation itself, and finally back to the meeting room for an evaluation of the experience and mutual reinforcement for success. Like other methods in this approach, the specific activities of clients and group worker vary from phase to phase in treatment. If the group is to succeed attention must also be paid to the group variables which either impede or enhance the progress of treatment. The procedure may be the major intervention strategy or may be used in combination with a variety of other procedures for attaining and maintaining the remediation of agoraphobia and other complaints the client brings to the treatment situation. For those group workers who work with clients with inordinate fears, especially agoraphobia, this is a method, by virtue of its empirical support, meriting extensive consideration.

REFERENCES

Emmelkamp, P. M G (1982) *Phobic and obsessive-compulsive disorders Theory, research and practice*, Plenum Press: New York.

Emmelkamp, P. G , & Kuipers, A. (1979) Agoraphobia. A follow-up study four years after treatment. *British Journal of Psychiatry*, *134*, 352-355.

Emmelkamp, P. G., & Kuipers, A. (1985). Behavior group therapy for anxiety disorders, in Upper, D. and Ross, S. M., *Handbook of Behavior Group Therapy*, New York: Plenum Press, 443-472.

Emmelkamp, P. G. & Mersch, P. P. (1982). Cognition and Exposure in Vivo in the Treatment of Agoraphobia Short-Term and Delayed Effects, *Cognitive Therapy and Research*, *6*(1), 77-88.

Foa, E. B., Jameson, J. S., Turner, R. M., & Payne, L. L. (1980). Massed vs. spaced exposure sessions in the treatment of agoraphobia. *Behaviour Research and Therapy*, *18*, 333-338.

Goldstein, A. J., & Chambless, D. L. (1978). A reanalysis of agoraphobia. *Behavior Therapy*, *9*, 47-59.

Gustavson, B., Jansson, J., Jerremalm, A., & Ost, L. (1985). Therapist Behavior During Exposure Treatment of Agoraphobia. *Behavior Modification*, *9* (4), 491-504.

Hafner, R. J., & Marks, I. M. (1976). Exposure in vivo of agoraphobics. Contributions of diazepam, group exposure, and anxiety evocation. *Psychological Medicine*.

Hand, I., Lamontagne, Y., & Marks, I. (1974). Group exposure (flooding) in vivo for agoraphobics. *British Journal of Psychiatry*, *124*, 588-602.

Jansson, L., Jerremalm, A. & Ost, L. (1984). Maintenance Procedures in the Behavioral Treatment of Agoraphobia. A program and some Data. *British Association for Behavioral Psychotherapy*.

Kanter, N. J., & Goldfried, M R. (1979). Relative effectiveness of rational restructuring and self-control desensitization in the reduction of interpersonal anxiety. *Behavior Therapy*, *10*, 472-490.

Marks, I. M. (1969). *Fears and phobias*. New York: Academic Press.

Marks, I M. (1970). Agoraphobic syndrome (phobic anxiety state). *Archives of General Psychiatry*, *23*, 538-553.

Mathews, Andrew M., Gelder, Michael G., & Johnston, Derek W. (1981). *Agoraphobia Nature and Treatment*, New York: The Guilford Press.

Rose, S. D. & Edleson, J. (1987). *Working with children and adolescents in Groups*, San Francisco: Jossey-Bass.

Sinnott, A., Jones, R. B., Scott-Fordham, A., & Woodward, R (1981) Augmentation of in vivo exposure treatment for agoraphobia by the formation of neighbourhood self-help groups. *Behaviour Research and Therapy*, *19*, 539-547.

Stamm, J. L Infantile trauma, narcissistic injury, and agoraphobia (1972). *Psychiatric Quarterly*, *46*, 254-272.

Teasdale, J. D., Walsh, P. A., Lancashire, M., & Mathews, A. M. (1977). Group exposure for agoraphobics A replication study. *British Journal of Psychiatry*, *130*, 186-193.

Telch, Michael J., Agras, W. Stewart, Taylor, C. Barr, Roth, Walton T., & Gallen, Christopher C. (1985). Combined Pharmacological and Behavioral Treatment for Agoraphobia, *Behavioral Research therapy*, *23* (3), 325-335.

Watson, J. P., Mullet, G E., & Pillay, H. (1973). The effects of prolonged exposure to phobic situations upon agoraphobic patients treated in groups *Behaviour Research and Therapy, 11*, 531-545.

Wolpe, J. (1973). *The practice of behavior therapy*, New York Pergamon Press.

Zitrin, C. M., Klein, D. F., Lindemann, C., Tobak, P., Rock, M., Kaplan, J H., & Ganz, V. H (1976). Comparison of short-term treatment regimens in phobic patients. A preliminary report. In R. L. Spitzer & D F. Klein (Eds). *Evaluation of psychological therapies*, Baltimore. John Hopkins University Press.

An Adaptive Approach to Group Therapy for the Chronic Patient

Louise M. Camblin
Walter N. Stone
Linda C. Merritt

SUMMARY. This paper presents a model for group treatment with chronic mentally ill patients. In this approach the therapist focuses on members' adaptive capacities and encourages problem solving. Interventions recognize but do not explore affects. The therapist does not pursue transference reactions but attempts to remain within the patients' metaphors which are seen as efforts to deal with feelings inside and outside of their therapy setting. Through successful "action" patients build a sense of mastering problems and being helpful to one another. Potentially this increases self-esteem and enhances the patients' lives within the community.

The delivery of therapeutic services to the chronic patient in all forms has been neglected. Indeed, Lamb (1979) has wondered how could "professionals with a major responsibility for the fate of the mentally ill be so insensitive to the needs of their charges, not once, but repeatedly?" As a partial remedy, group psychotherapy may be an optimal treatment modality since members are provided help in overcoming difficulties in interpersonal relations, an antidote to social isolation, and support in the need for continuing medication.

Louise M. Camblin, MSW, ACSW, Walter N. Stone, MD, and Linda C. Merritt, MSW are from the Forensic Division of Central Psychiatric Clinic and the Department of Psychiatry, University of Cincinnati College of Medicine Correspondence may be addressed to Louise M. Camblin, Court Psychiatric Center, 222 E. Central Parkway—307 A, Cincinnati, OH 45202 The authors wish to thank the following individuals for their helpful suggestions in the preparation of this manuscript Robert L. Kunkel, J Scott Rutan, and Esther G. Stone.

Despite these rather specific therapeutic attributes, this approach also has been underutilized.

The chronically ill patients generally are less concerned with mental health issues than they are with psychosocial needs. When placed in the context of daily living, the needs for housing, food, clothing, transportation, and general medical care take precedence over emotional needs. In describing these patients, Chacko, Adams, and Gomez (1985) state:

> Often they come to treatment only when they face a crisis or an emergency, and even then, they do not come voluntarily, but are brought in by relatives, neighbors, or the police. They are more interested in survival than they are in self realization or self understanding.

The problem of a comprehensive and broad based care is further complicated by the reductionistic approach of many community mental health centers where the focus is almost exclusively on pharmacotherapy of the patient's disorder.

If the patient can be engaged in treatment, the work is a long term proposition, punctuated by crises superimposed on serious difficulties in forming satisfactory and reciprocal interpersonal relationships. Yet recent findings demonstrate that over extended time periods significant improvement, and perhaps even recovery may take place (Harding, Brooks et al., 1987). In part the problem lies with continuity of care, and in part with a lack of conceptual clarity regarding the appropriate and productive treatment strategies. Generally treatment for the chronic patient has been described as supportive therapy, a loosely defined term that may carry with it negative images for the therapist (Winston, Pinsker, and McCullough, 1986; Buckley, 1986). There has been a consequent tendency to assign patients requiring these services to the least experienced members of the therapeutic team, which further diminishes the likelihood of sophisticated therapeutic intervention.

Despite these general trends there have been efforts to define the goals and techniques of supportive therapy. This paper will selectively review the literature on the outcome and dynamics of groups with chronic patients. This will be followed by a description of our approach to group psychotherapy and an illustrative session. It is our goal to illustrate an adaptive strategy that can be utilized to develop a positive therapeutic engagement with these needy but difficult patients.

While outcome studies are limited, there is evidence favoring group versus individual treatment for the chronically ill. Shattan, Decamp, Fujii et al. (1966) and Prince, Ackerman, Carter et al. (1977) reported significantly reduced rehospitalization rates in aftercare populations who participated in group treatment. In contrast, O'Brien, Hamm, Ray et al. (1972) did not find a difference in rehospitalization rates. However, they found increased social effectiveness in group therapy participants when compared to those in individual treatment. Group therapy also increased patients' abilities to self-observe and allowed them to develop a feeling of belonging (Claghorn, Johnstone, Cook et al., 1974; Herz, Spitzer, Gibbon et al., 1974). Other benefits from group treatment are reduction of anxiety, enhanced communication skills and improved reality testing (Schultz and Ross, 1955). Thus, although the data have limitations, they support the use of group treatment as an effective and valuable aftercare strategy.

Little has been written about the dynamics of aftercare groups. Some authors have focused on the importance of group cohesion (Masnick, Bucci, Isenberg et al., 1971; Grotjahn and Kline, 1979; Rosen and Spitz, 1979), where the task of the therapist is to promote interaction, and help patients share with one another. Kanas, DiLella and Jones (1984), studying the content of the first 26 sessions of a group composed of discharged schizophrenic patients, support this clinical impression. The most frequent topics were encouragement of contact with others, and reality testing followed by expression of emotions, and advice giving. The authors suggest that this stratification of topics created a safe treatment environment.

Payn (1965, 1974) conceives of the therapeutic process as follows:

> The therapist discovers the group theme, verbalizes that theme for the group and through that process helps the patients feel understood. A successful session pulls members out of their isolation, gets them talking to one another, allows them to

> express feelings and helps them modulate inappropriate feelings and alter inappropriate behaviors.

Katz (1983) focuses on the value of metaphors in group treatment. He suggests that the therapist avoid interpreting the group themes directly, but views the metaphoric discussion as a "safe middle ground for both patients and staff members, between unacceptable, intolerable impulses and unproductive defensive operations." Lesser and Friedmann (1980), in a more ambitious view, believe that insight can be gained in aftercare groups. They note the emergence of recurrent group themes of separation-individuation, dependency, and abandonment. Avoiding these issues denies the patient an important growth experience, but the depth of the discussion should be controlled and the therapist should not personalize the transference.

The opposite view is put forth by Pattison, Brissenden, and Wohl (1967), and Yalom (1983) who found that schizophrenic patients respond negatively to groups that utilize insight oriented techniques. Kanas (1986), in a review of controlled studies of group therapy for schizophrenics, stresses that unconscious material should be avoided. Parloff (1986) in his discussion of Kanas' work points out the limitation of the studies and challenges clinicians and researchers to focus on the relatively new chronic population in the community and develop creative ways of adopting group treatment to that population.

In our work with groups of the chronic mentally ill the focus has been on enhancing living skills. Problem solving is a major issue with our groups. The problems emerge from the material presented by the patients, usually in the form of a group theme. Often this theme is related to the transference, which is understood, but not interpreted. Rather it is translated back into the metaphor or into the real world.

The recurrent themes at a reality level are concerned with housing, personal safety, money for food and transportation, and general medical care. Family relationships are seldom experienced as gratifying, rather they are sources of frustration and dissatisfaction. Full time employment is low priority, and only comes into focus when other issues have been addressed. These themes, generally, are expressed in dependency or hostility terms, with the hope, both overtly and covertly, that the therapist will be able to provide solutions. The therapeutic strategy is to engage patients in mutual problem solving, thereby expanding their ego capacities and increasing self esteem.

This article will describe the reaction of a group of chronic patients to a staff member's absence as well as a new clinic policy regarding financial interviews. These events are particularly stressful for those patients who often exhibit disruptive anxiety or maladaptive defenses to issues of dependency and separation. The session is chosen to illustrate our theoretical stance in working with chronic patients. It is presented to highlight an alternative to exploration of intrapsychic and interpersonal conflict or of transferences.

GROUP DESCRIPTION

The group had been in existence one and a half years at the time of this meeting. The members were selected from patients enrolled for treatment in a forensic clinic where they had been mandated by court order. Thus, in addition to the psychiatric diagnoses the patients had criminal records that ranged from misdemeanors, such as shoplifting, to felonies, such as gross sexual imposition. The psychiatric diagnoses included schizophrenia, affective disorders and personality disorders. Substance abuse problems were an additional element in these individuals' psychopathology. About 75% of the group members had prior hospitalization for mental illness. The ages of the participants ranged from 18 to 70 years; most were 20 to 30 years old. The patients were of low socioeconomic status. They did not have a sustained capacity to work or fill homemaker roles and generally were unemployed and supported through public assistance.

Patients were referred to the group following their initial evaluation or a period of individual treatment at the Court Psychiatric Center. None of the patients were in concurrent individual treatment, but individual appointments with the group therapists could be arranged as deemed necessary. The group met once weekly for one hour. The first 45 minutes of the session were lead by two clinical social workers. In the final 15 minutes a psychiatrist joined the group to evaluate and update the status of the patients' medications.

The group is labeled "Coffee Group." The co-leaders and members sit around a table. Instant coffee, sugar and cream are available in the room and the leaders bring in a small snack when the group begins. The census is 16 and weekly attendance varies from 3 to 12 members. Over time all members become acquainted with one another. The stated goals include helping patients increase social functioning and adaptation, decrease rehospitalization rates, and decrease criminal activity.

The members are free to speak about any topic they choose. The therapists try to encourage interaction, problem solving and reality testing, and generally eschew exploration of intragroup conflicts. Metaphors are understood within a psychodynamic perspective. Interventions are made within the metaphors and generally not translated in the transference, with the goal being to further the members' adaptive capacities, without overstimulating affects.

THE MEETING

The session was the first of two successive meetings when one of the leaders was to be absent on a previously announced vacation. Eight members were in attendance – four arrived before the session began, two entered with the leader, and two came approximately 15 minutes late. The leader opened the meeting by making two announcements. First she reminded the members that the other leader would be absent; second, she announced a new clinic policy that members would be required to undergo a financial interview. The leader added that because of their financial status it was unlikely that anyone would be required to pay for treatment.

Following the announcements Allen remarked, "There is no more sugar for the coffee." Others quickly followed wondering how all the sugar could have been used already. Several members suggested that perhaps some "outsiders" had entered the room and used the sugar. However, Barbara, who often assumed a leadership role, restated that the sugar was all gone and asked the leader to get some more. The therapist said that would not be possible since the session had already started. Barbara commented that sugar was available in the snack bar down the hall. She promptly left the room and returned in a few minutes with a handful of sugar packets which she shared with the group.

While Barbara was absent, Clara said that she was being pressured to place her elderly mother in a nursing home. She indicated that she was afraid to do this because she would be left without a means of support, since she shared her mother's Social Security benefits. The members asked Clara a number of questions trying to clarify the situation and seemed to be quite empathic with her dilemma. The leader commented that Clara was faced with a difficult decision and asked if other members could recall being in a similar situation of "having to make a big decision" and how they handled it. Allen stated that he just takes some action as he knows the problem won't go away by itself. The therapist then asked David, a young, mildly mentally retarded man, if he had any thoughts on this topic. He said that he had never had to make a big decision. Barbara, who had returned at this point, told him that he will have to before too long.

Barbara then began discussing her health problems and how her doctor cancelled her appointment and rescheduled it for the following week. She said that she felt disappointed but realized that she could wait another week to see her doctor. The members then began to discuss the problems they encountered when they tried to go to any of the specialty clinics at the city's public hospital. They talked about how crowded the clinics were and how long they had to wait to be seen. The leader commented on how frustrating that must be, to feel ignored and to wait so long for care.

In response to this intervention the group then returned to Clara's problem with her mother. Clara said that a worker from the Adult Protective Services was going to take her to apply for Social Security, but she didn't think that she would qualify. Barbara said that Clara should tell Social Security that she attends the group meetings and a report could be sent from the clinic to verify it. The leader acknowledged that was true. Clara stated that she was too embarrassed to tell the worker that she was receiving treatment at the Court Clinic as that information would reveal that she had been arrested. Many members shared their humiliation about their arrests, but concluded that almost everyone needs support sometimes, and that to get help for whatever reason should not be embarrassing. Members then provided constructive information on how to fill out the Social Security forms. With the time almost up and what seemed to be a partial resolution of the issue, the leader inquired if the silent members had anything to add. As planned, the psychiatrist then entered the room to discuss medications. Concurrently, the therapist spoke individually to several members regarding the need to complete the fee assessment forms.

DISCUSSION

This session illustrates the level of functioning that is possible in aftercare groups. The members are coping with two major stressors, the absence of one of the leaders, and to an equal extent, the anxiety created by a new clinic policy requiring fee interviews. The members managed their anxiety through metaphoric discussion and concomitantly dealt adaptively with some real, every day problems.

The initial topic of insufficient sugar signals a control theme and reflects the members' feelings about the absent leader and the impact of the new regulations which are experienced as a loss of nurturance. The belief that outsiders had come and taken the sugar highlights the members' feeling of being "ripped off," and refers not only to being short one leader, but the sense that the group boundaries cannot be protected by the leadership; i.e., they may have to pay a fee (Rice and Rutan, 1981). The leader did not encourage exploration of anger at this point. This strategy is concordant with Kanas' (1985) suggestion that direct expression or exploration of anger often is counterproductive by raising anxiety to levels that lead to regression or more primitive behavioral solutions. Barbara continued the theme by directly asking the leader to act. The leader's response was primarily a reminder to the members of her commitment to tasks within the room. This response seemed to enable Barbara (as the group representative) to mobilize herself, not remain helpless, and gratify the members' needs by getting the sugar.

This action must be distinguished from acting out. In an optimal situation patients would have the capacity for delay of gratification and be able to explore their feelings, including frustration and anger at the leader. The leader did not pursue these feelings nor did the members. Instead by getting the sugar Barbara both highlights the leader's limitations and simultaneously problem solves. It would have been less adaptive to remain in the room and continue to complain to the leader or to withdraw. As Katz (1983) has succinctly stated, "Feelings of helplessness were generally converted to those of effectiveness and competence: powerlessness was converted to mastery and control; overwhelming anxiety was converted to feelings of warm satisfaction at the successful completion of a task." Barbara set a proactive tone that was repeated later in the session.

The discussion that took place during Barbara's absence was about Clara being left without a means of support if she placed her mother in a nursing home. The context suggested that Clara was referring both to emotional and financial support. These elements were mirrored in the transference in relation to the forthcoming financial interview and the absent therapist. The therapist chose to focus on the "big decision" that overtly remained in tune with Clara's inner world, and is therapeutically neutral, enabling the members to find whatever solution works best for them. It demonstrates respect for members and their ability to help problem solve.

Allen stated an adaptive position in the context of Barbara's behavior by commenting that when faced with a difficult problem, you have to act because the problem won't go away by itself. This position was reinforced by Barbara's response to David and, moreover, she nicely distinguished between when one might delay and when action was appropriate. Implicitly she indicates an ability to handle some affects which is a sign of increasing ego capacities.

Apparently, the progressive step of taking responsibility evoked anxiety, since the topic shifted to the members' feelings regarding problems in trying to obtain care at the public hospital. The therapist's recognition of their frustration seemed to reverse this regressive response, and reestablished the problem solving mode. That culminated in the encouragement of Clara to expose the information that she was in therapy and had been arrested in order to pursue application for Social Security benefits. In addition, the therapist could support Clara's position with a necessary letter.

This session highlights the therapeutic benefits in pursuing an adaptive response. The therapist chose not to focus on frustration and anger which was felt to be counter productive instead she was quite content to focus on problem solving. If successful, this stance could lead to increased self-esteem and a firmer base from which the members could approach more difficult affect laden issues.

Often, group members are more familiar with survival strategies than the middle class therapist. They are able to help one another negotiate welfare systems and other problems in daily living (Stone, 1983). In this way, the group situation builds members' competencies in problem solving skills. As Payn (1974) notes, advice is often more acceptable when it comes from a fellow group member than when it comes from a leader, and the advice giver feels a sense of pride at being helpful.

Working through Clara's problem of a potential financial and emotional support allowed the group members to gain practical information about government assistance programs and ways to negotiate these systems. Barbara's suggestions were accepted by the group and she was acknowledged for her expertise. Barbara's history is of having been a high functioning individual prior to a psychotic break, and since that time she has felt denigrated by her family and friends. The group offers her a place where she can share with others, and have her suggestions considered and often appreciated. Overall, group members see that they are not helpless. When one group member is able to solve a problem, the other group members feel a sense of accomplishment at having been part of the process.

In a framework that emphasizes problem solving, patients may attend to painful affects. Members discussed the embarrassment of being arrested and coming to the clinic. Through their discussion they conclude that to come for help is positive and that they can manage their embarrassment about their acts and their needs. In this way they illustrate some growth as they are not overwhelmed by their feelings, but are able to proceed in an adaptive fashion. In the future, as members gain greater sense of self-esteem through adaptive problem solving, they might again be steered in the direction of dealing with more difficult feelings in the transference, either to the therapist, peers or to the clinic system.

CONCLUSIONS

The session is used to illustrate a productive group session with aftercare patients. While the goals of such groups often seem modest; e.g., increased socialization, cooperative problem solving, and modulation of powerful affects through verbalization, these are important issues in the everyday lives of chronically ill individuals. The therapist who has a broad based understanding of group dynamics is in a better position to foster growth at whatever pace these patients can manage.

Treatment of this population is particularly difficult and taxing since in our view it requires that the therapist recognize the group-as-a-whole dynamics, understand the level of group functioning which often includes use of metaphors, and then intervene at the most useful level. The task is complicated by the ever present survival and daily living issues that are used to convey messages to the therapist. Premature or ill-timed interventions focusing on the within group dymanics rather than remaining at metaphoric or reality level often lead to group fragmentation. In contrast more felicitous interventions at the proper level allow members to utilize their limited, potentially expandable skills in problem solving. Such a stance is both respectful and growth producing.

REFERENCES

Lamb, R. (1979) Roots of neglect of the long term mentally ill. *Psychiatry*. 42: 201-207.

Chacko, R.C , Adams, G.L., and Gomez, E. (1985) The care of the chronic mental patient A historical perspective. In Chacko, R.C. (ed) *The Chronic Mental Patient in a Community Context*. Washington, D.C. American Psychiatric Press.

Harding, C.M , Brooks, G.W., Ashikaga, T., Strauss, J.S., and Breier, A. (1987) The Vermont longitudinal study of persons with severe mental illness, II: long-term outcome of subjects who retrospectively met DSM III criteria for Schizophrenia. *American Journal of Psychiatry*. 144 727-735.

Winston, A., Pinsker, H., and McCullough, L. (1986) A review of supportive psychotherapy. *Hospital and Community Psychiatry*. 37. 1105-1114.

Buckley, P. (1986) Supportive psychotherapy A neglected treatment *Psychiatric Annals*. 16 515-521.

Shattan, S.P., Decamp, L., Fujii, E., Fross, G.G., and Wolff, R.J. (1966) Group treatment of conditionally discharged patients in a mental health clinic. *American Journal of Psychiatry* 122· 798-804.

Prince, R.M., Ackerman, R.E. Carter, N.C., and Harrison, A. (1977) Group aftercare: impact on a state-wide program. *Diseases of the Nervous System*. 38· 793-796.

O'Brien, C.P., Hamm, K.B., Ray, B.A., and Pierce, J.F. Luborsky, L. and Mintz, J. (1972) Group vs. individual psychotherapy with schizophrenics. *Archives of General Psychiatry*. 27: 474-478.

Claghorn, J.L., Johnstone, E.E., Cook, T.H., and Itschner, L. (1974) Group therapy and maintenance treatment of schizophrenics. *Archives of General Psychiatry*. 31: 361-365.

Herz, M.L., Spitzer, R.L., Gibbon, M., Greenspan, K., and Reibel, S. (1974) Individual versus group aftercare treatment. *American Journal of Psychiatry*. 313· 808-812.

Schultz, I.M., and Ross, D. (1955) Group psychotherapy with psychotics in partial remission. *Psychiatric Quarterly*. 29 273-279.

Masnick, R., Bucci, L., Isenberg, D., and Normand, W (1971) "Coffee and . . ."· a way to treat the untreatable. *American Journal of Psychiatry*. 128. 164-169.

Grotjahn, M., and Kline, F. (1979) Group therapy in psychiatric hospitals and outpatient clinics. In L.R. Wolberg and M. L. Aronson (eds) *Group Therapy 1979: An overview*. New York· Stratton Intercontinental Medical Book Corporation, pp. 111-116.

Rosen, A., and Spitz, H.I. (1979) The role of videotape in group psychotherapy with psychotic patient populations. *Group*. 3 213-228.

Kanas, N., DiLella, V.J., Jones, J. (1984) Process and content in an outpatient schizophrenic group. *Group*. 8· 13-20.

Payn, S.B. (1965) Group methods in the pharmacotherapy of chronic psychotic patients. *Psychiatric Quarterly*. 39· 258-263.

Payn, S.B. (1974) Reaching chronic schizophrenic patients with group pharmacotherapy. *International Journal of Group Psychotherapy*. 24· 25-31.

Lesser, I.M., and Friedmann, C.T.H. (1980) Beyond medication group therapy for the chronic psychiatric patient. *International Journal of Group Psychotherapy*. 30: 187-199

Katz, G. (1983) The noninterpretation of metaphors in psychiatric hospital groups. *International Journal of Group Psychotherapy*. 33 53-67.

Pattison, E M., Brissenden, A., and Wohl, T. (1967) Assessing specific effects of inpatient group psychotherapy. *International Journal of Group Psychotherapy*. 17. 283-297.

Yalom, I.D. (1983) *Inpatient Group Psychotherapy*. New York Basic Books.

Kanas, N. (1986) Group Therapy with Schizophrenics A Review of Controlled Studies. *International Journal of Group Psychotherapy*. 36 339-351.

Parloff, M.B. (1986) Discussion of "Group Therapy with Schizophrenics." *International Journal of Group Psychotherapy*. 36: 353-360.

Rice, C.A., and Rutan, J.S. (1981) Boundary maintenance in inpatient therapy groups. *International Journal of Group Psychotherapy*. 31: 297-309.
Kanas, N. (1985) Inpatient and outpatient group therapy for schizophrenic patients. *American Journal of Psychotherapy*. 39: 431-439.
Stone, W.N. (1983) Some dynamics of children's participation in aftercare groups. *International Journal of Group Psychotherapy*. 33: 333-348.

New Directions in Children's Group Therapy: Integrating Family and Group Perspectives in the Treatment of At Risk Children and Families

Gerald Schamess

SUMMARY. This paper examines the clinical observation that children's therapy groups are most effective when they are constructed to symbolically represent functional family systems. The interrelationship between psychodynamic/developmental theory as it is applied to group treatment with children and family systems theory is discussed in the context of two intervention projects; a genogram group for latency age children who were living in families that had been disrupted by separation and/or divorce, and a mother-child group for single teenage mothers and their infants or toddlers. Both of these programs were designed to serve client populations that find it difficult to participate in more traditional forms of social work treatment, and both are based on the principle that children's groups can be constructed to planfully address and modify dysfunctional family structures as well as intra-psychic and interpersonal difficulties.

This paper will describe two projects in which family oriented treatment techniques were adapted for use in developmentally oriented children's therapy groups. The decision to combine family and group procedures was made with the aim of developing treatment models that would simultaneously (or at least sequentially) address deficits in ego organization and also directly influence dys-

---

Gerald Schamess, MSS, is Professor at Smith College School for Social Work.

functional family structures. These projects reflect an ongoing interest in finding innovative ways of working with clients who are difficult to engage in treatment and/or who do not respond positively to traditional therapeutic technique. The first project was designed to reduce confusion about family composition and structure and at the same time, promote progressive emotional development in latency age children suffering from somatoform disorders (DSM IIIR 300.00 and 300.70), as well as a wide range of serious behavioral, interpersonal and academic problems. All of the children in this group came from disengaged families (Minuchin, 1974) which had been disrupted and reconstituted with disheartening frequency. The second project, a mother/infant/toddler group, was organized to help single teenage mothers and their children deal more adaptively with the vicissitudes of attachment, separation and individuation. Since both mothers and children in this population are thought to be "at risk," the group was also designed to support the mothers' attempts to master adolescent life stage tasks and establish functional intergenerational roles and boundaries in the new families they had created.

Traditional models of children's group therapy have been well described by at least three generations of theorist/practitioners, including (by generation), Slavson (1943); Hallowitz (1951), MacLennan (1977), Rosenthal (1977), Scheidlinger (1960) and Schiffer (1969); Azima (1986), Frank (1983), Kraft (1986), Reister and Dies (1986), Schamess (1986) and Soo (1986). Even though these models are usually conceptualized in psychodynamic/developmental terms, all of them employ a therapeutic approach which implicitly recognizes the role that pathogenic family interactions and internalized object relations play in both the etiology and treatment of childhood psychopathology. Treatment theory is based on a set of implicit principles which describe the group as a symbolic family and suggest that corrective responses to family reenactments are at the core of the treatment process. From this perspective children's therapy groups are viewed as constructed representations of functional family systems in which the members reenact "unacceptable" feelings and perceived pathogenic (dysfunctional) relationships as part of the group process. In the following section I will examine some of these principles and discuss their application to both the genogram and the mother/infant/toddler groups.

The concepts presented in this paper are derived from drive theory, object relations theory and family systems theory. Although these are competing frameworks they share a number of important ideas in common, the most compelling of which, from a clinical standpoint, is that children internalize representations of individual family members and of their family systems-as-a-whole. These internalized representations provide a basis for reenactments of symptomatic family relationships with individuals and groups in the community at large. Reenactments reflect unconsciously determined attempts to master traumatic experiences and/or establish secure (previously known) and predictable relationships with peers and caregivers outside the family. The processes outlined above can be explained theoretically as projective identifications, transference displacements, manifestations of the repetition compulsion or reflections of dysfunctional family roles and structures. Over and above their connection to particular theoretical frameworks, these explanations attempt to provide a context for understanding clinical interactions in which the boundaries between self and object become fluid as children attempt to master problematic introjects and dysfunctional family relationships. This way of thinking is particularly important for therapists who treat children individually or who view treatment from an intrapsychic perspective. It suggests that the holding environment which develops in treatment is populated not only by the real child-therapist dyad and the transferential child-therapist dyad, but also by mental representations of all the other significant members of the child's family, however that family is constituted.

If we take this formulation seriously, it supports the idea that all child treatment should be viewed from at least two different perspectives; first as an attempt to modify intrapsychic structures and internalized object relations and second, as a form of family therapy. There is a good deal of clinical evidence to support the view that when children succeed in achieving higher levels of ego integration they also succeed in modifying the symptomatic roles they had previously played within their family systems. There is also evidence that symptomatic children who are not able to change the roles they play in their family systems or the personal meanings they construct in trying to understand those roles, usually do not achieve lasting intrapsychic change. From this perspective, the crucial therapeutic issue is not whether therapists provide individual, group or family treatment, but whether they recognize that, at one level of meaning, the transferences which unfold during treatment reflect family roles and structures as well as problematic relationships with individual caregivers and internalized object relations. Enactments and reenactments occur regardless of whether family roles and relationships are reproduced symbolically as a function of the transference relationship, or through direct interaction in the presence of a therapist, with family members who actively contribute to the child's emotional difficulties.

To the best of my knowledge, no one has yet attempted to compare children's group and family therapy in terms of the assumptions they make about how treatment works. While a systematic comparison is beyond the scope of this paper, it is worth noting that the modalities share some important ideas in common about the nature of practice (Durkin, 1981). Both theories emphasize that children change when they have an opportunity to: (1) experience, (2) enact (or reenact) and (3) reconsider the ways in which they ordinarily function within their family systems. The theories further state that when these enactments or reenactments evoke corrective, interpersonal responses from significant others, children respond by developing more adaptive coping strategies both inside and outside their family systems. In processing these corrective interactions children recognize that the roles they ordinarily play in relation to family members (or people who, in their minds, represent family members) are personally dysfunctional and that there are other ways of relating to significant others which are much less problematic. Within constructed groups of unrelated participants, realizations of this kind occur as a result of transferential (symbolic) interactions. Within already established family systems, they result from interactive initiatives that can only be accommodated through structural change in already established family roles.

Psychodynamically oriented therapists explain treatment by saying that children's therapy groups provide a holding environment in which the members experience periods of controlled regression and reintegration. During these periods the therapist unconditionally accepts feelings, wishes and needs which are rooted in early developmental fixations, while at the same time, helping the group-as-a-whole contain or limit problematic behaviors. In this formulation, it is assumed that changes in intrapsychic functioning result from corrective interpersonal interactions which serve as the basis for new, more adaptive identifications.

From a family systems perspective the curative elements in children's group therapy are also understandable in terms of symbolically charged interactions with peers and adults. Over time, group members develop new interpersonal skills and coping strategies and, in doing so, alter previously established symptomatic roles and relationships. They then transfer these new skills and expectations from the group to their families where they attempt to modify the personally dysfunctional, but homeostatically important roles they had previously played. The process is quite efficient when other family members are able and willing to alter established family structures. Behavioral change occurs first within the group and then within the family system and is viewed as a necessary precondition for change in the individual's self-system; i.e., self-concept, object relations, ego functioning, etc. This analysis suggests that among its other characteristics, children's group therapy is a form of family oriented treatment conducted with groups of unrelated individuals.

Psychodynamic and systemic explanations differ significantly in regard to the relative weight they assign to feelings, impulses, internalized object relations and intrapsychic structures on the one hand, and family roles, interpersonal interactions, the homeostatic requirements of family systems and behavioral change, on the other. Nonetheless, they share a compelling vision that experientially based interpersonal learning within a family or family-like context is fundamental to the therapeutic process. In considering the similarities and differences between the theories, I am impressed by the degree to which they complement each other. Since one emphasizes the intrapsychic aspects of treatment and the other emphasizes the interpersonal/systemic aspects, when combined, they provide a much fuller description of the treatment process then either model provides separately. The substantive areas of disagreement concern the optimal unit of treatment (i.e., real families or symbolic families) and how therapeutic interventions can best be sequenced (i.e., should therapy attempt to alter family roles and relationships as a necessary precondition for modifying affective states and intrapsychic structures, or vice versa?). To borrow a concept from Gestalt psychology, even though the controversies are substantive, the essential differences are about what constitutes "figure" and what constitutes "ground."

Without attempting to resolve the controversies it seems important to emphasize that children's therapy groups have always been constructed with the aim of modifying both ego functioning and family relationships. Although the family oriented aspects of the modality have not been emphasized in the literature, they are nonetheless, fundamental to treatment. Along with most other psychodynamically oriented clinicians, children's group therapists generally assume that by modifying drive organization, ego functioning and object relations, treatment will also modify family roles and relationships. More specifically however, children's group therapists establish and maintain a family focus by constructing groups that simulate functional family systems. These created family systems provide the medium through which change takes place.

There are at least two basic reasons for organizing treatment along these lines. The first is that the mental life of children is inextricably intertwined with the mental life of significant family members, particularly caregivers. To paraphrase Winicott, there is no child without a family (or some substitute caregiving system). Most therapists agree that children can only be treated in conjunction with one or more of their caregivers, and/or through the creation of symbolic relationships which facilitate reenactments of problematic family roles and relationships within the therapeutic process. Children's groups that simulate functional family systems always meet at least one of these criteria even when parents are not treated concurrently.

The second reason is based on the observation that the families in which children grow up are the first groups to which they belong. Normative developmental processes create early associative connections between family life and group life which influence the perceptions, expectations and behaviors that children bring to all their other group experiences. This is to say that children recreate important aspects of their family roles and relationships wherever they go. When therapists are attuned to this tendency, they are more likely to understand the displaced and projected family dramas which unfold in groups as treatment progresses. By constructing groups in ways that accentuate the tendency, group therapists can reverse the process through which experiences are transferred from family to group life and thereby influence the family systems in which dysfunctional roles and relationships originally developed.

These observations provide a sound rationale for constructing children's groups to simulate functional family systems. Unfortunately however, children's groups do not automatically shape themselves into functional symbolic families. Providing a corrective experience for children who come from different kinds of family systems and who function at different stages of psychosexual development, requires both flexibility and careful planning (Schamess, 1986). In traditionally organized children's therapy groups, therapists evoke mental representations of symbolic families by creating an emotional environment which encourages the reenactment of symptomatic family roles and pathogenic experiences with primary caregivers as part of the group process. In order to set the stage for these reenactments, the therapist performs a number of prosaic tasks which predictably evoke images of family life. These include, (1) preparing the group room before every session and partially cleaning it as each session ends, (2) providing craft materials and activities that, given the members' age and level of intrapsychic organization, are not only interesting and appealing, but also encourage self-expression, (3) offering advice and concrete help to group members who want and need assistance (or contact with a caregiver), (4) encouraging independence in group members who want and need to function more autonomously (or need to distance themselves from a caregiver), and (5) shopping for, preparing and serving a snack which the members are encouraged but are required to eat, family style, with the therapist.

Simply by performing these "housekeeping" functions, children's group therapists assume many of the roles that parents ordinarily play within functional family systems. This role specific behavior encourages group members to relate to the therapist as if s/he is a symbolic parent and to the group-as-a-whole, as if it is a family system; both similar to and different from their own family systems. The therapist further enhances these images by presenting him/herself as an emotionally available, empathetic caregiver who unconditionally accepts problematic feelings and behaviors. By modelling adaptive behaviors and attitudes, therapists encourage the members to identify with the problem solving techniques, expressions of competence and mastery, and manifestations of affective responsiveness which they embody. Group members identify with their group therapists for precisely the same reasons they identify with their parents; i.e., because the therapists model attitudes and behaviors which the members experience as both need gratifying and admirable.

By highlighting the transference reenactments which emerge when children participate in constructed family systems, I have expanded the traditional explanatory paradigm for children's group therapy. While retaining many of the original drive theory formulations, I have added concepts drawn from object relations theory and family systems theory. Based on my clinical experience, the expanded paradigm is preferable because; (1) it more accurately describes how treatment actually works in children's therapy groups and (2) it provides a set of guiding principles which encourage clinically sound experimentation with new techniques and new models of intervention that address the needs of children with serious emotional problems (Scheidlinger, 1960; Trafimow and Pattak, 1981).

My interest in constructing children's groups that directly influence family roles and relationships is based on attempts to treat and/or supervise the treatment of children living in extremely dysfunctional family systems. Initiating and maintaining treatment with such children is difficult if not impossible, when parents are unable or unwilling to be treated concurrently. Parents seem to be "uncooperative" (i.e., self-protective in ways that are problematic for their children and/or the children's therapists) when they feel so vulnerable emotionally that they cannot tolerate any examination of their own feelings and relationships, and/or when their living situations are so stressful that they can only attend to their children's maturational needs and experiences intermittently, on the rare occasions when the environmental stressors temporarily abate. Those of us who are committed to treating children who are seriously "at risk," have to explore creative ways of intervening sensitively and effectively in family systems even when parents are not available for and/or amenable to traditional forms of individual, group or family treatment.

At this point in time I have identified two ways of modifing traditional forms of children's group therapy so that they more directly address problematic family roles and relationships. The first of these involves constructing multi-family groups that focus on mother/child dyads as the sub-systems most amenable to change. This method works particularly well with mothers and their first or second born children, six years old or younger. Such groups permit children to play and interact freely with each other under the guidance of a therapist or developmentally oriented early childhood educator while their mothers meet separately to discuss feelings and issues that are of concern to them. The children's and mothers' groups meet separately in adjacent spaces with the understanding that each group's boundaries are semi-permeable. Once these conditions have been established, the parallel groups interact in ways that directly influence family relationships and structures as well as individual functioning. Several practitioners have written about using groups of this kind to educate mothers about child development and/or to promote more constructive relationships between mothers and their young children (Holman, 1979; Phillips, 1985; and Bittner, 1984).

The second option involves using a medium of communication which makes it possible for the members of traditionally organized children's groups to; (1) understand how their family systems are constructed and (2) deal more adaptively with the personally dysfunctional but homeostatically important roles they are expected to play within their family systems. Genograms serve this purpose extremely well. This approach to treatment is particularly effective with older latency age children who are already symptomatic and whose parents are not available for concurrent treatment. The group process encourages the members to modify those aspects of their family relationships over which they have some control and to make peace with those aspects they cannot change. Mary Wagner (1988) notes that "what children can't change, they have to learn to live with." She goes on to say that children will find relatively constructive ways of dealing with problematic family situations when they are helped to recognize and acknowledge the roles and relationships they would like to change. They will only begin to accept that they are not responsible for their family's problems and also that they are not inherently defective as human beings, after they have actively tried to change those problematic relationships (with help from a therapist) and discovered that their parents cannot change.

The genogram group which will be described directly below, encouraged children to learn about how their families are constructed, why the families had evolved in particular ways and what roles they were expected to play in relation to other family members. As a result of this process, the group members became more "realistic" about their relationships with other family members, an accomplishment which allowed them to modify some of the dysfunctional roles they had previously played both at home and at school.

The mother/infant/toddler groups that will be described toward the end of the paper, provided the therapists with an opportunity to intervene both therapeutically and preventively during the transitional period when single teenage mothers were leaving their families of origin to create new family systems of their own. These multi-family groups were quite effective in controlling the intergenerational transmission of psychopathology from one family system to another and in helping the group members develop more satisfying (and healthier) relationships with their children then they had experienced with their parents.

THE GENOGRAM GROUP

The ten and eleven-year-old children selected for this group were fourth and fifth grade students in a small rural public school located in Western Massachusetts. The boys and girls who participated were originally identified by the school nurse/psychologist as children who visited her office three or more times a week for the treatment of minor physical complaints (cuts, scrapes, aches, pains, nausea, running noses, tiredness, etc.). For the most part these complaints were psychosomatic in origin. Their trips to the nurse's office seemed motivated by a wish for care and attention, as well as by a defensive need to avoid stressful situations both at home and at school. Teachers, administrators and guidance counsellors had previously identified these children as problematic. All of them had serious behavioral, social and/or academic problems which made them notably dysfunctional at school. Further evaluation revealed a pervasive pattern of serious family disruption. Divorce, separation, remarriage, a variety of reconstituted family systems, foster care and adoption were commonplace realities in these children's lives. The group met once a week for thirty sessions. It was co-led by the nurse/psychologist who had originally identified the children and the social worker who provided therapeutic services for the school system (Davis, Geike and Schamess, 1988).

In considering how they might construct a group that would address these problems the leaders remembered Yalom's (1984) observation that therapeutic groups should make feelings, thoughts and memories which had previously been unconscious, "visible," both to the individual group members and to the group as a whole. This observation led to the realization that genograms could provide a tangible medium for helping children visualize complex family relationships which they did not understand, either for defensive or developmental reasons. The leaders hypothesized that the orderly presentation and elaboration of each member's genogram would create an arena of group interaction that was sufficiently distant from problematic family interactions to make group members feel relatively safe, but was also evocative enough to stimulate progressive disclosure of important memories and feelings at a pace that would be emotionally tolerable.

Since the act of drawing a genogram is intellectually challenging to latency age children, it not only supports phase specific cognitive growth, but also creates a certain protective distance between any given description of family fragmentation and the intense affects associated with fragmentation as an actual event. By focusing on one child's genogram at a time and limiting the amount of time spent drawing and discussing each child's genogram, the leaders successfully controlled the level of anxiety that emerged as group members revealed painful experiences. These structural constraints allowed the members to develop some understanding of and enthusiasm for the process and, over time, facilitated a successful resolution of their internal struggles around trust and self-revelation. For the children in this group, learning to draw their genograms without help from the leaders also promoted a sense of competence and accomplishment that visibly enhanced their self-esteem.

Group Structure and Boundaries

The group met once a week for sixty minutes at a public elementary school in Western Massachusetts. There were five members, three boys (S., D., and T.) and two girls, (B. and J.), ages nine to ten (grades four and five). All five of the children who were originally invited participated actively in the group. One of the boys (T.) moved away from the community after the twelfth session. The other four members participated for the entire thirty sessions. Attendance was close to perfect and the children were quite enthusiastic about their participation in the group.

The first fifteen minutes of each session were taken up by one member working on his or her genogram. Since this included the therapists, each child had an opportunity to work on his family every eighth session (five children and two therapists). We made it clear that during the opening fifteen-minute segment, when a genogram was being presented, we expected all members to participate in the process. Everyone was free to ask questions and make comments and over time, everyone did. Initially, and for some time thereafter, the therapists would draw the member's genograms. When individual members felt more comfortable with the process they began to add their own information as they revealed it.

When the fifteen-minute presentation and discussion of a genogram was finished, the presenter decided what activity the group would undertake for the next thirty-five minutes. The group members were quick to pick up on the time sequence and were adamant in their adherence to the schedule. Clearly the play period offered considerable relief from the tension of the first fifteen minutes.

Following the activity there was a ten-minute snack period. The snack consisted of peanut butter or cheese and crackers, milk or juice, and was provided by the therapists. We felt that by providing food for the group we were emphasizing our willingness and ability to care for the members. In addition, the snack provided some badly needed oral gratification as well as a feeling of emotional security.

Sitting around the table created a family like atmosphere which encouraged the group members to talk together in a relaxed and companionable way.

There was no room for flexibility in this structure, and any rules that the leaders or the group members felt were needed had to be established within the framework. Over time we began to think of the structure as a kind of ritual which sequentially involved working, playing, and sharing a meal together. Each part of the ritual was constructed to provide opportunities for individuality, cooperation, and group cohesiveness. Each child had an opportunity to be special, but always as an integral part of the group as a symbolic family. The group was organized so that the most important therapeutic work would be accomplished as members presented and discussed their genograms; that is, as they came to better understand how their families were constructed and how they had been affected by changing family systems.

Group Process: Genograms

Over the course of the group, members became increasingly interested in presenting and elaborating on their own and other member's genograms. Initially they had to learn the mechanics of doing a genogram, a task which was challenging but manageable with help from the therapists. For this reason, there was not much discussion of the genograms drawn during the first round of presentations. Because the pace was slow, members had an opportunity to test out how revelations about their families would be received by the group as a whole. As individual members felt that their stories were accepted, the group became increasingly cohesive.

Over time, group members began to inquire about specific aspects of one another's families. Their inquiries gradually became more searching and more sensitive to the needs and feelings of other members. The questions that individual children provided gave us an opportunity to observe where each child might be defending against feelings and memories related to his or her own family situation. The leaders were careful to note each child's questions and to explore those questions when the child who asked them next presented his/her genogram.

After each person had presented his/her genogram three times and there was no additional information to add or questions to ask, the leaders began to hold sessions with all the genograms tacked on the walls together (sessions 22-30). During these group meetings all of the group members shared and reviewed their histories together, making comparisons, discussing similarities and differences in their backgrounds, talking about changes, and identifying new ways of coping with fragmented family situations.

Process: Activity Period

As the group matured, the members gradually began to talk about family issues during the activity period. This was especially true when the chosen activity was the "Talking Feeling and Doing Game." Over time the leaders altered the prescribed format of the game to facilitate discussion. For those not familiar with the game, a brief explanation will be helpful. Normally, a child lands on a colored space and draws a card from the color deck. S/he reads the question out loud and if the question is answered, gets a chip. The turn then moves to the next child. The questions are designed to probe for intrapsychic and interpersonal material. Because the goal was to encourage the group members to talk about themselves and their families, the leaders encouraged the group to discuss each question by inviting all of the members to say how they would have responded. The members were not required to respond, but since responses were encouraged, they came to be expected. This technique not only encouraged individual children to talk but also led to a sharing of ideas and feelings between group members, and thus greatly enhanced group cohesion.

During the middle phase of the group, as the members played the "Thinking, Feeling, Doing" game, they began to acknowledge that their responses to the game cards were elaborations of the memories, fears and wishes they had presented and discussed earlier in the session when they were drawing their genograms. Statements such as "I go along with you guys about feelings about parents not taking care of kids" (J.). "My real father gave me up" (S.), and "What would make me happiest is if my mother loved me" (J.), were heard at these times. In response to one card, a group member

(D.), revealed his anxiety about an impending change in family relationships. He commented that his father's live-in girl friend was okay as a girl friend, but would be intolerable as a step-mother.

Process: Snack

As noted earlier, a ten-minute snack period always followed the activity. The snack was provided by the therapists, who also served it during the early sessions of the group. Midway through the group, on their own initiative, the children assumed more responsibility for serving. Shortly thereafter, the members joined together in saying that they wanted to provide the snack on a rotating basis. They were quite insistent about doing this. The leaders were surprised by the initiative and after some private discussion outside the group, decided that the request reflected the members' difficulty in relying on adults (in this instance, the therapists) for basic nurturance. For that reason their suggestion was politely refused. The leaders allowed the members to serve but not to provide the food, since they didn't want to reinforce the members' tendency to assume parental roles. During the course of this discussion one of the group members (D.) reported how, when he visited his mother, he would take his allowance with him so he could buy groceries for her. In passing, he also mentioned that he would get up early in the morning to make them both breakfast, even though his mother frequently slept until noon. In this instance, it was clear that he was taking care of his mother as he wished his mother would take care of him. His comments reinforced our decision to continue providing the snack.

Over time, the snack period turned toward a discussion of family matters in much the way the activity period had. Before each session the therapists would hang up the genogram of the child who was scheduled to present that day. During the last phase of the group, all of the diagrams remained on the wall for everyone to view throughout the entire session. When the group settled down for snack, it was easy and natural to reflect on the genograms since they surrounded us. It was not unusual for a group member to spontaneously make additions to his/her genogram during snack. Near the end of one session, a group member (J.) suddenly jumped up, ran to her genogram and added a name to a man's place. It was a poignant moment when she announced that she finally knew her father's name. Another group member (S.) demonstrated the lack of continuity in his relationships when he looked at one of the therapist's genograms which showed a ten-year-old adopted daughter. He asked, "Do you still have her?" When the therapist said "yes," he seemed dumfounded. It was hard for him to believe that an adoptive parent would care for a child for so many years. S.'s subsequent comments made it clear that this interaction had alleviated some of his anxiety about being abandoned by his new foster father because of his provocative (testing) behavior.

Outcome

The four children who completed the group all showed notable improvement. On their graduation from elementary school there were no reports of academic, social or behavioral problems. In addition their psychosomatic illnesses had all but disappeared. For the most part, the group members did not visit the nurse/psychologist at her office and on the rare occasions when they did, they came to talk about issues that were emotionally distressing to them. Informal follow-up contacts with school personnel confirmed that they all had made satisfactory adjustments to junior high school and that their overall functioning was well within the normative range. Follow-up contacts with parents or other caregivers indicated that there had been marked improvement at home.

The treatment process in this group can be briefly summarized by focusing on the brief vignettes that describe "D's" participation. At the time he was referred, his teachers described him as "very frustrated and angry . . . completely unable to accept criticism of any kind." He had come close to failing several subjects and had also been the object of repeated disciplinary action (visits to the principal's office, notes home, etc.). He visited the nurse/psychologist's office several times a week with a variety of vague somatic complaints. In outlining his genogram he revealed that he was living with his father and that his mother and father were divorced. Over time he added that his mother had been neglectful of him before the divorce and also had a history of alcoholism and emotional disturbance. He visited her regularly on weekends. As this material emerged, he initiated the idea that the group members should take turns providing snack for the group. When the leaders politely turned down his suggestion, "D" argued and then became pensive. Sometime later, he remarked in passing, that he regularly used his allowance to buy groceries for his mother because he was concerned about her health. The group members expressed surprise about this practice, another response which had the effect of making "D" thoughtful. He later talked about how unhappy he was with the woman his father was planning to marry. As the group progressed he gradually seemed to resolve his conflict about whether he could be loyal to his mother and still have some positive interest in his father's fiancée. Although he continued to visit his mother regularly, his need to take care of her diminished and he was able to talk directly about how disappointed he was with her when she slept all morning while he was visiting.

During the course of treatment he progressed from a cognitive description of his family organization, to a transference reenactment (his wish to buy food for the group in much the way he regularly bought food for his mother), to a direct expression of his conflictual feelings about attachment and loyalty, and finally to a more adaptive resolution of his conflict. These changes were accompanied by an increased capacity to acknowledge and verbalize his angry and sad feelings toward both his mother and father. In addition, as his relationship with his biological mother became more "realistic," he was also able to develop a stronger alliance with his father and begin the process of forming an attachment to his perspective step-mother. This progression reflects structural change in "D's" extended family system, as well as markedly improved ego functioning.

GROUPS FOR MOTHER/CHILD DYADS

Mother/infant/toddler groups (Schamess, 1987, 1989) are the primary treatment modality in an agency based pregnancy and parenting program for single teenage mothers and their children. Shortly after giving birth, mothers who are thought to be emotionally "at risk" are invited to attend a group which meets weekly at the local family agency. They are told that child care will be provided and are encouraged to bring their infants to the agency with them. The groups are designed to meet the psychosocial needs of young women who suffer from moderate to severe emotional dysfunction. Initially, members look to the groups for emotional support, education, environmental assistance and guidance in caring for their children. Over time, however, they begin to talk more directly about the feelings and problems that are of most concern to them and the groups begin to focus on treatment issues. The group leaders encourage most of these young mothers to participate in the program, with their children, for two or more years. An extended period of treatment is necessary both to help them deal with phase specific developmental issues and to internalize the therapeutic gains they have made.

Initially, the newborn infants may be cared for by their mothers as they talk together in the mother's group room, or by a developmentally oriented nursery school teacher who takes care of the infants in the adjoining children's group room. The connecting door between the rooms remains open until the children no longer need to touch base with their mothers during the hour and a half group sessions. Given normative developmental processes, this usually takes about two years. During the first two years of treatment the mothers are always in a position to observe (and hopefully, identify with) the teacher's way of working with their children. Mothers and children also interact as they arrive at and leave the Agency together. As children progress through the differentiating and practicing subphases of separation-individuation (Mahler, 1975), the teacher works toward helping them separate physically and emotionally from their mothers. Within the children's group they are encouraged to interact freely with one another and to make use of the developmentally oriented play equipment that is set out in the room.

The parallel mother/infant/toddler groups function simultaneously at three levels of meaning and experience; first, as normative, developmentally oriented play groups for children, second, as experientially oriented treatment groups for mothers, and third, as multifamily groups in which mother/child dyads regularly interact as family systems or sub-systems, depending on whether the newly created families include the child's father or another man with whom the mother is living. These interacting therapeutic processes are illustrated in the following summary. The themes to be discussed are typical of themes that emerge in all of these groups during the second year of treatment.

As children enter the rapprochement subphase of separation-individuation, the mothers' irritation and impatience with them increases markedly. The toddlers' entry into rapprochement coincides with the mothers' attempt to deal more adaptively with their own unresolved issues about separation-individuation; i.e., do they want to leave their parents' homes to live on their own, can they finish their high school degrees, can they learn how to drive, what will it be like to care for their children while trying to work, how can they find a man who will love them, will they be able to control their tendency to abuse both drugs and alcohol? In trying to deal with these phase specific developmental issues, the mothers frequently feel trapped, angry and hopeless about their future prospects. Typically, their own high levels of anxiety make them at least somewhat unsympathetic to the children's need for care and reassurance about the mothers' emotional availability at times of need. If the therapists try to reassure the mothers that their children's anxious demandingness is related to normative developmental processes and therefore will pass in time, the mothers, in typical adolescent fashion, usually remain adamant. They insist that the children are "bad" and need "discipline" because they constantly interfere with the mothers' activities both at home and in the group.

The mothers enacted this theme in treatment by arriving at the Agency, and literally pushing their children into the adjacent group room even when the children were unwilling to separate. During group sessions, the mothers reiterated the message that the children were a bother by insisting that they stay in their group room whether they wanted to or not. When children visited the mothers to talk or make physical contact, the mothers glanced at them, listened briefly and/or hugged them distractedly, and then insisted that they return to their own room. If the children were reluctant to go, the mothers scolded, yelled, threatened and at times, "swatted" them to make them "behave." Although the nursery school teacher had been working consistently with the children to help them separate and enjoy the children's group, she found it very difficult to manage five or six children who had literally been pushed, crying into the group room.

At this point it is worth emphasizing that I am not describing these interactions in order to criticize the mothers. In fact, the mothers were doing their very best under extremely difficult circumstances. As adolescents, they had an understandable need to talk about their own wishes, needs and feelings without being constantly interrupted. For the mother child dyads in this group, rapprochement was a developmental phase during which the mothers' needs and the children's needs were not in synchrony. Describing the process is relevant because it indicates the degree to which mothers and children were struggling with similar psychological issues, although at very different levels of development.

As noted above, the group leaders first attempted to deal with the problem by explaining the children's need for contact and initiating a discussion about better ways of calming children who are distressed about separation. The mothers responded first by insisting that their children were "bad," and then by visibly trying to suppress the irritation that this attempt at "guidance" evoked. For brief periods of time they did their best to follow the therapists' suggestions, but then, inevitably, they would lose patience again. It soon became clear that their cognitive progresses could not contain the intense affects and impulses that dealing with separation issues engendered. When the leaders decided that group members were "swatting" their children too often, they established a "no swatting" rule in the group and suggested that the mothers apply the rule at home also. The therapists thought the members would be relieved by the rule and over time, discovered that they had, indeed, been relieved. However, their immediate reaction at the level of manifest content, was to become furious. They accused the therapists of making a "big deal" out of nothing, of siding with the children against them and of talking to them in the same way their parents did. The therapists explained their role as mandated reporters, empathized with how difficult it is to think about what children need when their own needs are so intense, and stuck to their guns about "no swatting" in the group, ever. As this process evolved over time, the therapists realized that, while the mothers were yelling more at them, they were yelling less at their children.

Eventually the mothers revenged themselves on the therapists with considerable imagination and delight. On leaving a group session (obviously having planned this in advance), they stood in the parking lot, shouting up through the open windows for the leaders and everyone else in the Agency to hear: "We're out here in the parking lot beating up our children and there isn't a thing you can do about it." Since the Agency's child welfare orientation was well known to the group members, they were fully aware of how hostile and provocative they were being. On returning to the next group session, they were eager to know how the group leaders had responded. When the group leaders indicated that they viewed the incident as a rather funny prank, but that they also understood how angry the mothers were feeling toward them and how frustrated they were feeling toward their children, the mothers began to talk more openly about how difficult it was to care for their children and build an independent life for themselves at the same time. They went on to talk about how little confidence their own mothers have in them, even now, and about how angry they are that their parents didn't stop them from doing things that eventually got them into serious trouble. One member summed up the group's feelings by saying, "People who don't protect you, don't care about you."

As the furor died down, it became clear that the mothers had viewed the limits as protective. After expressing their transferential anger toward the therapists and having it accepted, they were much better able to deal with the children's separation anxiety and demandingness, both in the group and at home. They also began to talk quite openly about times when they felt like neglecting and/or abusing the children and about their efforts to manage their "frustrations" more constructively. As many other therapists have observed, the more they talked about these impulses, the less they acted on them.

While the major therapeutic work was done in the mothers' group, the children's participation in a parallel group not only precipitated the developmental issues and made them visible, but also kept them alive as an essential part of the group process long enough for the mothers to resolve them. Eventually, of course, the children benefited as much from the therapeutic process as the mothers did. After the crisis was resolved the mothers were not only better attuned to the children's phase specific developmental needs, but were also able to help the children participate in a group of their own which over time, became an enjoyable growth enhancing experience. In looking at the program's overall effect, it seems clear that the parallel mother/child, multifamily groups; (1) enhanced the children's capacity to deal with the sub-phases of separation-individuation, (2) made it possible for the mothers to reenact and work through their ambivalent feelings toward their own mothers and (3) markedly reduced the intergenerational transmission of psychopathology from the mother/grandmother dyads to the mother/child dyads. While only time will tell whether these new family structures are stable, the mother/childs group were certainly helpful in reducing serious levels of phase-specific conflict between these teenage mothers and their young children.

CONCLUSION

This paper expands the traditional explanatory paradigm for children's group therapy by including concepts drawn from object relations and family systems theory. The aim is to encourage practitioners to think about children's therapy groups as constructed symbolic family systems in which corrective, transferentially charged interactions provide the major impetus for growth and change. This view suggests that children's therapy groups can be organized to address deficits in ego organization and dysfunctional family structures within a single treatment framework. It also provides a set of functional guidelines that can be used to facilitate the construction of groups for specific populations of "at risk" children whose parents are not available for traditional forms of concurrent treatment. Two examples of specialized children's groups are presented; the genogram group for symptomatic latency age children and the mother/infant/toddler, multi-family group for psychologically dysfunctional single teenage mothers and their newborn infants or toddlers.

The use of genograms as a primary medium of communication

encourages children to review, reexperience and redefine their relationships with parents and other members of their primary and extended families. This occurs within the context of a growth promoting, normative peer group experience which encourages the development of age-appropriate social skills and relationships. Group members alternate between periods of carefully structured regression, intellectual exploration and cognitive-emotional reorganization. The process of presenting and discussing individual genograms allows them to reexperience the disruption of their family units and to grieve for distant or absent family members, as well as for the loss of their idealized fantasies about how family life "ought to be." By talking openly about changing family structures, the members begin to accept that other children have also suffered significant losses, that it is not necessary for them to feel stigmatized by their own losses and that as individuals, they are not responsible for the breakup of their family units. The method is particularly useful because it encourages children to construct new meaning systems that help them understand their relationships with significant family members. As they learn to view their families more "realistically" group members gradually find ways of modifying the dysfunctional roles they had previously played without endangering and/or disrupting their primary relationships.

The parallel mother/child group format for mothers, infants and toddlers provides a structured opportunity for mothers to reexperience and rework issues involving attachment and differentiation at the same time their children are experiencing them for the first time. As the mothers interact with and care for their infants and toddlers, their own needs for nurture as well as their problematic experiences with primary caretakers are reenacted in the immediacy of a shared group experience where the needs can be understood and worked through. At the deepest level of unconscious representation, it seems likely that the mother/infant groups represent a nurturant, protective mother. At the level of current reality however, peer and therapist expectations encourage both mothers and children to work toward more adequate levels of adaptive functioning. The interplay between mothers' and children's groups enables the mothers to construct new family systems that are more functional than the systems they grew up in, thus interrupting the intergenerational transmission of psychopathology from one family system to the next. Simultaneously, the children's groups support and enhance normative developmental processes and in doing so, serve an important preventative function.

REFERENCES

Aichhorn, A. (1935). *Wayward Youth*. New York· Viking Press.

Axline, M. (1947). *Play Therapy*. Boston Houghton Mifflin.

Azima, F.J.C. (1986). Countertransference: In and Beyond Child Group Psychotherapy. in *Child Group Psychotherapy Future Tense*. Reister A.E. and Kraft, I. (Eds.), Madison, Conn.· International Universities Press, 139-156

Bittner, R. (1984). Therapeutic Mother-Child Groups A Developmental Approach. *Social Casework* 65·3; 154-161.

Davis, L., Geike, G. & Schamess, G. (1988). The Use of Genograms in a Group for Latency Age Children. *International Journal of Group Psychotherapy* 38, 2, 189-210.

Durkin, J. (1981). *The Living Group Psychotherapy and General Systems Theory*. New York· Brunner/Mazel, Inc.

Epstein, N. & Altman, S. (1972). Experiences in Converting an Activity Group into Verbal Group Therapy. *International Journal of Group Psychotherapy* 22 93.

Frank, M. (1983). Modified Activity Group Therapy with Ego Impoverished Children. in *Ego and Self Psychology*. Buchholz, E.S. and Mishne, J.M. (Eds.), New York Jason Aronson, p 145-156

Gabriel, B. (1939). An Experiment in Group Treatment. *American Journal Orthopsychiatry* 9 146.

Ganter, G., Yeakel, M. & Polansky, N (1967) *Retrieval from Limbo*. New York· Child Welfare League of America.

Ginott, H. (1961). *Group Psychotherapy with Children*. New York McGraw-Hill

Hallowitz, E. (1951). Activity Group Therapy As Preparation for Individual Treatment. *International Journal of Group Psychotherapy* 1 4,337.

Holman, S.L. (1979) An Early Intervention Program for Developmentally At-Risk Toddlers and Their Mothers. *Clinical Social Work Journal* 7 3, 167-181.

King, C. (1959). Activity Group Therapy with Some Schizophrenics. *International Journal of Group Psychotherapy* 9·184

Kraft, I. (1967). Group Therapy in *The Comprehensive Textbook of Psychiatry*. Freedman A and Kaplan, H.I. (Eds.), Baltimore, Md. Williams and Wilkins.

______ (1986). Innovative and Creative Approaches in Child Group Psychotherapy. in *Child Group Psychotherapy, Future Tense*. A.E. Reister and I. Kraft (Eds.), Madison, Conn. International Universities Press.

Lifton, N. and Smolen, E. (1966). Group Psychotherapy with Schizophrenic Children. *International Journal of Group Psychotherapy* 16: 23-41.

MacLennan, B. (1977). Modifications of Activity Group Therapy for Children. *International Journal of Group Psychotherapy* 27. 85-96.

Mahler, M., Pine, F. & Bergman, A. (1975). *The Psychological Birth of the Human Infant*. New York: Basic Books.

Minuchin, S. (1974). *Families and Family Therapy*. Cambridge· Harvard University Press

Phillips, N.K. (1985). Mother-Child Interaction Group, Model for Joint Treatment. *Social Casework* 66 2; 91-97.

Redl, F. & Wineman, D. (1951). *Children Who Hate*. Glencoe, Ill · Free Press.

Reister, A.E. & Dies, R.R. (1986). Research on Child Group Therapy: Present Status and Future Directions. In *Child Group Psychotherapy, Future Tense*. Madison, Conn. International University Press, 173-222.

Rosenthal, L (1977). Qualifications and Tasks of the Group Therapist with Children. *Clinical Social Work Journal* 5·191-199.

Schamess, G. (1986). Differential Diagnosis and Group Structure in the Outpatient Treatment of Latency Age Children. In *Child Group Psychotherapy Future Tense*. Madison, Conn. International University Press, 29-70.

______ (1987) Parallel Mother/Infant/Toddler Groups A Developmentally Oriented Intervention Programme for Unmarried Teenage Mothers. *Journal of Social Work Practice* 2:4, 29-48.

______ (1989). The Group as Transitional Object In *The Expanding World of Psychodynamic Group Therapy*. S. Tuttman, (Ed.), Madison, Conn.· International Universities Press (In Press).

Scheidlinger, S. (1960). Experimental Group Treatment of Severely Deprived Latency Age Children. *American Journal Orthopsychiatry* 30:356-368.

______ (1965). Three Approaches with Socially Deprived Latency Age Children. *International Journal of Group Psychotherapy* 15 434-445.

Schiffer, M (1969). *The Therapeutic Play Group*. New York. Grune and Stratton

Schiffer, M.S. (1984). *Children's Group Therapy. Methods and Case Histories*. New York The Free Press.

Slavson, S.R. (1943). *The Therapeutic Play Group*. New York· Grune and Stratton.

Soo, E. (1974). The Impact of Activity Group Therapy Upon a Highly Constricted Child *International Journal of Group Psychotherapy* 24: 207-216.

______ (1986) Training and Supervision in Child and Adolescent Group Psychotherapy In *Child Group Psychotherapy Future Tense*. Madison, Conn. International University Press, 29-70.

Speers, R and Lansing, C. (1965). *Group Therapy in Childhood Psychoses*. Chapel Hill, N.C. University of North Carolina Press.

Sugar, M. (1974). Interpretive Group Psychotherapy with Latency Age Children. In *Journal of the American Academy of Child Psychiatry* 13: 4.648-666.

Trafimow, E. & Pattak, S. (1981). Group Psychotherapy and Objectal Developmental in Children. *International Journal of Group Psychotherapy* 31: 193-204.

______ (1982). Group Treatment of Primitively Fixated Children. *International Journal of Group Psychotherapy* 32: 445-452.

Wagner, M. (1988). Personal Communication.

Yalom, I. (1984). Personal Communication.

The Discharge Issues Group: A Model for Acute Psychiatric Inpatient Units

Keith Armstrong

SUMMARY. The topic of discharge from inpatient psychiatric units is written about frequently. However, inpatient groups which focus on discharge issues are rarely discussed. This paper briefly reviews the literature on discharge issues groups with the finding that while long-term psychiatric units focus on patients' feelings about leaving the hospital, existing acute adult psychiatric unit groups do not. An alternative model, the Discharge Issues Group, which does allow for patients to express their feelings about discharge, is presented. Two case examples are cited to illustrate how the group functions.

INTRODUCTION

Planning for discharge is an essential component of patient hospitalization. In a library search of 359 articles written about discharge issues in the ten years from 1975 to 1985, only five discussed the concept of a discharge planning group (Batey, 1980; Burrows, 1985; Heine, 1975; Ledbetter & Batey, 1981; Zabusky & Kymissis, 1983). Of the groups described, three addressed the discharge needs of adults on an acute inpatient unit. Two of these articles emphasized teaching patients about various resources while the third had a task-oriented approach (Batey, 1980; Heine, 1975; Ledbetter & Batey; 1981). Of the other two articles (Burrows, 1985; Zabusky &

Keith Armstrong, MSW, is the psychiatric inpatient social worker at the Veterans Administration Medical Center, 4150 Clement Street, San Francisco, CA 94121. He acknowledges Anne Cook, OTR, and Joan Liaschenko, RN, for their contributions to this paper.

Kymissis, 1983), one described a discharge group on a long-term psychiatric unit in England while the other article described a discharge issues group for adolescents.

The focus of the discharge group in two articles by Batey (1980, 1981) is a "consumer education model which emphasizes the individual's responsibility in discharge planning" (Ledbetter & Batey, p. 417). In this model, a multidisciplinary team, consisting of a social worker, a vocational rehabilitation specialist and a pharmacist, presents inpatients with information about various aspects of treatment. The clinical pharmacist advises about medications, the social worker discusses appropriate housing, and the vocational rehabilitation specialist provides and coordinates "services to assist the individual in obtaining or returning to gainful employment" (p. 418). The resource group begins in the early stages of hospitalization. Patients attend the voluntary group twice a week for an average of six times. The group is used in conjunction with a partial hospitalization program for patients who choose to utilize these services after discharge.

Heine (1975) writes about the discharge group she leads called the Daily Living Group. The focus of the group is on transition planning. The objectives of this structured, task-oriented group are (1) to give information and (2) to provide a forum to discuss patients' progress and feelings about their discharge plans. For example, a patient might express his concern about applying for work through role playing a job interview. However, Heine does not process patients' feelings about separating from the hospital. The group meets twice a week for one hour. Each patient attends an average of five sessions.

Two long-term inpatient groups which address patients' feelings about leaving the hospital are outlined below. Burrows (1985) writes about a "Leavers" group designed to facilitate transfer from a long-term hospital setting to a short-term transition unit. The goal of this group is "to develop insight into the problems of leaving and answer them with a problem-solving approach" (p. 41). For example, one of the goals addressed by the group is to provide a trusting and supportive atmosphere in which patients can learn ways of coping with being labeled mentally ill. The group meets twice a week for thirty-five minutes. Patients attend an average of 15 times.

Zabusky's (1983) adolescent group focuses on aiding in the resolution of identity conflicts and assisting in the transition from the hospital to placement in the community. This is accomplished through role playing upcoming interviews and discussing feelings about issues such as separation from families and fears about leaving the hospital. The group, which averages five members per session, meets once a week for 30-40 minutes.

In this article we discuss the importance of an inpatient discharge group which focuses on feelings of patients. Many times patients have difficulties saying goodbye to staff members, other patients, and the institution. Our group helps patients face the sometimes painful process of termination. Although research has yet to be conducted, we believe that addressing the patients' concerns about leaving the institution can positively affect their transition and may lengthen their stay in the community.

THE DISCHARGE ISSUES GROUP

The Discharge Issues Group we facilitate takes place on the Psychiatric Inpatient Unit of the San Francisco Veterans Administration Medical Center. This is a 28-bed, unlocked ward serving veterans with a variety of diagnoses. The unit is comprised predominantly of men, ages 20 to 80. All patients are voluntary members of the unit and must not pose any imminent danger to themselves or others. The average length of stay is about three weeks. Patients who are in the discharge phase of treatment attend the group. Those patients who are disruptive, very disorganized or severely brain-damaged do not attend (Yalom, 1983). The group is not mandatory but is strongly endorsed by the treatment team. Referrals occur in four ways: (1) group leader recommendation, (2) primary therapist recommendation, (3) multidisciplinary team recommendation, and (4) patient self-referral. The group meets once a week for an hour, and its size varies from four to nine patients. The average number of sessions attended is three. The group is led by the staff social worker and the occupational therapist or clinical nurse specialist.

The objectives of the Discharge Issues Group are:

1. To create a safe environment for patients to discuss their fears, anxieties, and hopes regarding their impending separation from the hospital. Time is allotted for patients to discuss termination concerns with group leaders and patients.
2. To provide opportunities to give and receive information (patient-patient, staff-patient, and patient-staff) (Batey, 1980; Ledbetter & Batey, 1981).
3. To assist patients with taking responsibility for their discharge (Buckwalter & Kerfoot, 1982).
4. To decrease patients' sense of isolation through the sharing of experiences in group (Kanas, 1985).
5. To help patients reflect on their treatment, noting gains and areas of weakness (Burrows, 1985).

Many patients come from environments in which they are independent adults struggling to provide food, clothing and shelter for themselves. When admitted to the Psychiatric Inpatient Unit they are immediately immersed in a community which provides them with both physical and psychological care. It is no wonder that in this environment patients become both dependent and close to each other and staff. Acknowledging this experience and focusing on terminating from other patients, staff, and the institution assists patients in ending their hospital stay. As they discuss their concerns about leaving, patients begin to address issues which may cause problems after discharge. The group setting enables patients to support each other's transition from the hospital to the community.

The group begins five minutes after the hour. The door is closed, signaling that group is in session. Late-comers are not allowed to enter because of the need to quickly develop a cohesive group. They are approached after the group by one of the group leaders to discuss their reasons for being late and their current discharge plans. Each group session is viewed as a separate, free-standing event with the therapists as active group leaders (Yalom, 1983).

Due to the patients' varying needs and abilities to tolerate stress, the group begins with a warm-up exercise which allows the members an opportunity to interact with each other prior to coming together in a circle as a group. Two examples in facilitating group process and creating cohesion are described below.

We have the patients break up into dyads to discuss pertinent issues about discharge. Subjects include patients' plans for follow-up treatment, living situation and use of leisure time. After ten minutes the group reconvenes, and members are asked by the therapists to present their partners' plans regarding discharge. This allows patients to talk intimately and listen to other members prior to the formation of a group circle.

Another exercise we have found useful is to have the leader write an unfinished statement on the blackboard (e.g., "I am concerned about ______ when I leave the hospital"), allowing the patients to free associate and complete the statement. Patients are allowed to respond as much as they like. One of the leaders writes the responses on the blackboard. After about ten minutes the group comes together to discuss the responses. Questions like, "Do the members see any patterns in these answers?" or "How do people feel about the responses?" help members talk about leaving the hospital. Often the responses are ambivalent: members are excited and happy about returning to the community but at the same time may be frightened and very sad.

Important themes will often emerge from the exercises which can be addressed in the group. One of the issues that frequently arises is saying goodbye. A patient in the group is asked to name another member of the inpatient community whom he/she will miss when he/she leaves the hospital. (This person may or may not be a member of the group.) The patient is then asked if he/she has thought about saying goodbye and is given the opportunity to actually say goodbye within the context of the group, or to role play saying goodbye to the absent inpatient community member. Afterwards, the patient is asked if it was hard to say goodbye. "What made it difficult? Did you say what you wanted to? What stopped you?" Other members are invited to comment on the patient's style of saying goodbye by responding to questions such as "Did it appear difficult for John to say goodbye? Will it be hard for you?"

Many other themes evolve from these exercises and can be addressed in the group. Topics which frequently emerge include:

1. Patients' dissatisfaction with their treatment, e.g., "I did not get what I needed."
2. Fear of the unknown, e.g., "I am frightened of the future."
3. Feelings of helplessness, e.g., "There is nothing I can do about my situation."
4. Concerns about placement, e.g., "I am worried about going to the board and care home."
5. Specific questions regarding concrete discharge issues, e.g., "How do I get on general assistance?"

Since each session is a freestanding and separate event, it is imperative to finish the work started in the group meeting. Patients should feel as if some of their concerns about leaving have been addressed and consequently they are prepared for discharge. Discharge is an inevitable experience for all members of an acute inpatient community. Sharing ways to cope with this often painful experience while preparing for transition into the community are the primary tasks of the Discharge Issues Group.

The following cases are typical examples of Psychiatric Inpatient Unit discharge issues.

Case No. 1: J.F. is a 61-year-old veteran with a history of schizophrenia coupled with intermittent panic attacks. He was evaluated by his day treatment coordinator and admitted to the Psychiatric Inpatient Unit due to his increasing anxiety and decreased ability to care for himself. In the past, the patient had lived in inexpensive hotels with one previous failed attempt at a board and care home.

> I always liked living on my own. That board and care home just didn't work out. The food was terrible and there were just too many people living there. I can't live in a hotel anymore. I get so scared . . . and then I hyperventilate.

It was evident to both leaders that J.F. would need to be involved in the Discharge Issues Group early in his hospital stay. The patient attended five sessions. He discussed past failures in both independent and supervised living situations, identifying potential problems that could arise. J.F. articulated his fears about leaving the hospital and discussed the progress he had made during hospitalization. Finally he was given the opportunity to say goodbye to staff and other patients. He talked about what he would remember most about his hospital stay, and he was given feedback by both patients and group leaders about his work. He was told he would be missed. J.F. subsequently made a successful transition to a new board and care home and continues to attend the day treatment center on a regular basis.

Case No. 2: B.D. is a 45-year-old veteran with a diagnosis of borderline personality disorder and substance abuse. He had been living alone in a hotel until a suicide gesture precipitated his admission to the Psychiatric Inpatient Unit. "Living in that area is too depressing. Drugs are too easy to get." During his hospitalization, B.D. was referred to a substance abuse halfway house but turned this down, citing "too many rules and regulations there. They don't want me to have contact with my best friend. I could never do that." The patient attended one Discharge Issues Group during his brief hospitalization. He was provided with a safe place to express his irritation at the "system" for "putting me right back in the same place as I was before." He was gently confronted by another patient who pointed out his refusal to attend the halfway house program. The patient continued to deny his responsibility in turning down the halfway house option, letting the therapists know he was not ready to hear this information. The group was able to address his feelings about leaving the hospital as well as his concern about returning to his downtown hotel. In addition, he was made aware of other members' concerns about leaving and consequently felt less alone. B.D. was provided with the opportunity to say goodbye to the other members of the group. During this process, other members showed concern about his discharge plans. The group members gave him feedback about his accomplishments on the unit. B.D. was discharged to a hotel and has recently been successful in obtaining full-time employment.

DISCUSSION

In every discharge group examined (Batey, 1980; Burrows, 1985; Heine, 1975; Ledbetter Batey, 1981; Zabusky & Kymissis, 1983), the social worker is one of the group leaders. He/she is vital to have as a group leader because of his/her skills in facilitating groups and knowledge of community resources. Co-leaders come from a number of disciplines, such as nursing, vocational rehabilitation, pharmacy, and occupational therapy. Since each profession brings specific knowledge to the group, it is important to use the knowledge base and refer to other disciplines in areas of uncertainty.

Our Discharge Issues Group is led by the social worker on the unit with the occupational therapist or clinical nurse specialist as the co-facilitator. Both the occupational therapist and the nurse can provide an illuminating perspective regarding the patients' day-to-day functioning on the psychiatric inpatient unit. Their knowledge about a patient's ability to care for him or herself is invaluable to the social worker in making appropriate discharge plans. This is particularly useful with those patients who are resistant to placement. For example, the group leaders can use the information provided by the occupational therapist or nurse to gently confront a patient's unrealistic plan to live independently. This knowledge base, coupled with an interest in learning group work, makes the occupational therapist or nurse an excellent choice as co-therapist.

The group serves patients with impending discharges in a variety of ways. It allows opportunities for group members to share information and feelings. Unlike other groups described above (Batey, 1980; Ledbetter & Batey, 1981), where members are recipients of information from professionals, our group addresses the emotional needs of patients as well.

Discharge issues groups always address future plans of patients. However, helping patients understand their inpatient experience and allowing them time to discuss feelings about leaving are techniques not emphasized in other adult acute inpatient groups. In his description of inpatient group work with adolescents, Zabusky (1983) writes that a number of issues, especially loss and separation, surface when patients are facing discharge from a psychiatric setting. It is also important for adults—with characterological impairments, or who are psychotic—to address loss and separation during their hospital stay. Helping patients begin this process is an important treatment focus which can continue in other psychotherapy groups, community meetings, and in individual work while the patient is still in the hospital. Hopefully, patients can utilize the experience of successfully separating from the hospital with future relationships that involve separation.

CONCLUSION

In this article we have presented a format for conducting a Discharge Issues Group. Our group attempts to provide a number of varied services to a diverse population. Helping patients discuss their concerns about leaving, talking about their future plans, and answering resource questions in a safe environment, create a successful group. As one patient stated, "This group is like a dress rehearsal for discharge. Without it, I would never think about what I am going to do when I leave." Very little has been written addressing discharge and the difficulties in leaving the secure environment provided by the hospital. Clearly, research needs to be conducted on the effectiveness of these groups. It is our belief that the Discharge Issues Group provides a vital link in the transition from the hospital to the community.

REFERENCES

Batey, S.R., Dees, A.C., and Ledbetter, J. Using a resource group to coordinate services in discharge planning. *Hospital and Community Psychiatry, 1980, 31, 417-418.*

Buckwalter, K and Kerfoot K. Teaching patients self care a critical aspect of psychiatric discharge planning. *Journal of Psychosocial Nursing Mental Health Service, 1982, 20, 10-15.*

Burrows, R. Group therapy. *Nursing Mirror, 1985, 160, 41-43.*

Heine, D. Daily living group *American Journal of Occupational Therapy, 1975, 29, 628-630*

Kanas, N. Inpatient and outpatient group therapy for schizophrenic patients. *American Journal of Psychotherapy, 1985, 39, 431-439.*

Ledbetter J and Batey, S R Consumer education in discharge planning for continuity of care *International Journal of Social Psychiatry, 1981, 27, 282-288*

Yalom, I. *Inpatient Group Psychotherapy, 1983.* NY Basic Books, Inc.

Zabusky, G. and Kymissis, P. Identity group therapy a transitional group for hospitalized adolescents. *International Journal of Group Psychotherapy, 1983, 81, 99-108.*

Short-Term Group Psychotherapy with the 'Family-Absent Father' in a Maximum Security Psychiatric Hospital

Deborah Wolozin
Edward Dalton

SUMMARY. This article describes a 10 session task focused group for mentally ill fathers in a forensic setting. The authors will describe group structure, group process and some effects of the therapy. Although these men are involuntarily hospitalized and thus separated from their families, their relationship with their children is an important one. The premise of this paper is that a focus on the father's role provides support and potential treatment opportunities for the fathers themselves.

REVIEW OF THE LITERATURE

There is little literature on the experience of the father who is incarcerated or hospitalized. Raubolt and Rachman (1980) in their writing about a therapeutic group experience for fathers note, "There is a need to delineate the role of the father in development and to develop treatment procedures that recognize, encourage and

---

Deborah Wolozin, LICSW, ACSW, and Edward Dalton, LICSW, ACSW, were clinical forensic social workers at the Institute of Law and Psychiatry, McLean Hospital, Belmont, MA at the time the group described in this paper was conducted. They both worked at Bridgewater State Hospital, Massachusetts' only maximum security psychiatric hospital. Address correspondence to Ms. Wolozin at Long Beach Reach, Inc., 26 West Park Avenue, Long Beach, NY 11561. This paper was presented at the 1986 annual meeting of the Parenting Symposium, in Philadelphia, PA.

support active fathering." Raubolt and Rachman's group members were middle income, professional men, but this need exists for the mentally ill, forensically hospitalized father as well. Fathers in a maximum security hospital may not be active in their child's upbringing in the same way as a father who is working and living with his child, but the work of the professional in a hospital setting can help the father to identify, understand and accept his particular part in his child's life.

When researchers study families of men who are hospitalized or imprisoned they commonly focus on the effect of this absence on the children. When therapeutic recommendations are made, treatment is suggested for the children themselves, rarely for the father. Biller (1981) cites numerous studies looking at the effects of father-absence on children's development. Father absence has often been linked with poor personal and social adjustment in the children left behind. Attention has also been focused on the degree to which the socioeconomic level of the family has been changed by the father's absence. Biller looks at father-absence in general, whereas other authors have focused on father-absence due specifically to incarceration. Sack, Seidler and Thomas (1976), Gamer and Schrader (1981), and Gamer and Gamer (1983) all look at the effects on children when the father is absent due to incarceration. These authors emphasize the importance of maintaining and strengthening family relationships when a parent is imprisoned. Strategies are suggested, such as providing support services, including the opportunity for regular visitation and involving the whole family in therapy where the impact of separation and the social pressures of incarceration can be discussed.

While these observations are significant, they appear to have overshadowed the emotional needs of the 'family-absent father', i.e., the father who is separated from his family. Little is written from the perspective of the father. What are the emotional strains that a father feels when he is without his family? What are his needs with respect to his children and family? Is the assumption that fathers do not have feelings about this? Traditionally, fathers are looked upon as irresponsible and uncaring for 'abandoning' their family, and not fulfilling the father's role. Less attention is paid to the psychological reasons that might compel a father to feel he must leave his family such as a father's belief that he could not fulfil his sense of the father's role as financial provider, family protector, or role model. There is also less interest in the psychological effects on the father of separation due to hospitalization or incarceration. The authors conjecture that some of this thinking, blaming the father, has seeped into what mental health professionals choose to address in therapy and in research.

There have been several attempts to work with incarcerated fathers. Marsh (1983) described a group led in a prison where parenting and communication were discussed. Communication, specifically, parents' commands and their childrens' compliance were measured before and after the group. Parents were able to use behavioral techniques to achieve a higher rate of compliance from their children leading to the subjective observation of "general improvement in the family harmony." At MCI-Norfolk, one of Massachusetts' medium security prisons, a group of incarcerated fathers found a way to communicate with their children about their lives in prison (1981). This group wrote and published a booklet entitled, *A Day in Time, A Day in Prison*, which describes prison life using language and descriptions that a 9-year-old child can understand. To quote the foreword in *A Day in Time, A Day in Prison*,

> We laid out our aims; . . . to allay the children's fear about the health and well-being of their fathers, . . . to help children understand that in spite of being in jail we still have the same feelings as do people outside and to describe some of the complex and confusing feelings that children may have toward the incarcerated parent.

The authors believe that in addition to helping their children, this booklet is an example of these men's attempts to order and understand their own fears and anxieties about prison life. In addition to providing a tool with which to communicate with their children, we believe that this process of identifying, understanding and accepting their situation helped to allay anxieties in the fathers themselves.

Yet another important aspect of work with forensic fathers is helping them to talk about the fathering they received. Fraiberg, Adelson and Shapiro (1975) note in their work with young mothers,

> In remembering, they are saved from the blind repetition of that morbid past. Through remembering they identify with an injured child (the childhood self), while the parent who does not remember may find himself in an unconscious alliance and identification with the fearsome figures of that past.

Fraiberg et al. and others point to the important work that must be done in helping mothers remember their own experiences with a parent. With necessary adjustments made for the limitations of a short-term group therapy, we have extended their work to fathers. This work of remembering can help a father to empathize with his child, and thereby avoid reliving his own painful childhood experiences through his own children.

Thus we have attempted in our group to tie these aspects together: remembering, support and education. By offering the forensic father an opportunity to talk about these issues, the leaders have acknowledged this powerful life role.

PRACTICE

This group was run on two separate occasions and consisted of 5 men who attended regularly for the 10 week term. In the first group one man declined to continue after the first session. In the second group, two men stopped participating after several sessions, one stating that he suffered heightened anxiety in the group and the other, that his hospital activity schedule prevented his participation. The patients' age range was from early twenties to mid-sixties. The age of patients' children ranged from infancy to early adulthood. These men suffered from a variety of psychotic and character disturbances. Patients were committed to the maximum security state hospital for civil and criminal reasons. Their legal histories ranged from minor aggressive behavior to murder. Contact with their children ranged from frequent visits by their children to no visits for extended periods of time. Patients were married, divorced and separated. Group therapy candidates were initially interviewed by the two group leaders to assess their interest and motivation. At that time family background information was reviewed. The group leaders also asked if the patient was receiving any other type of psychotherapy. No other selection criteria were used.

The group was a ten session, task focused group. The topics included family history, child development, communication with children, divorce and custody issues and parenting roles.

An identical questionnaire was administered in both the first and last sessions. This questionnaire was designed to aid men to focus their thoughts for the upcoming meetings as well as to provide some means for personal assessment of the benefits they received from the group discussions. In the questionnaire men were asked to identify problems with their children, describe their relationship to their children and their expectations for changes in their relationship with their children. After they had completed the questionnaire in the last meeting, the men were given their questionnaire from the first meeting to compare their responses.

Each session the leaders focused the group by presenting a task in the form of an open-ended sentence such as, "A happy time with my child(ren) was . . .," or a role playing activity such as a telephone call between father and child. On another occasion fathers were asked to tell a story about being with their fathers or persons that were like fathers to them. Responses to these tasks were the basis for that week's discussion.

Therapists used particular techniques because the group was time limited and focused. For example, leaders used a supportive technique, often generalizing issues among men without exploring issues related to individual pathology. Leaders took a round robin approach to ask each man to respond to the week's discussion. This task at times included setting limits on the more talkative members as well as encouraging the more withdrawn patients to share in the discussion. Leaders announced termination weekly because of its particular significance in a short term group.

The group leaders found that their leadership tasks were different with this group than with a more heterogenous inpatient group. Specifically, they spent less time redirecting members to the subject at hand and found men more spontaneously engaging with one another about the issues. Group leaders observed that the more regressed patients were included regularly in the group discussion. The leaders did not encourage group members to explore highly charged issues such as intense rage or incestuous relationships. The therapists did generalize and reframe issues to place them in the context of universal parenting issues for all fathers. They also made connections from week to week by reviewing the issues of the previous week during the first few minutes of each session. This provided continuity as well as informing members who had been absent the previous week of the past discussion.

There were several dominant themes discussed in these meetings. Men wondered how to maintain a relationship with their children while they were hospitalized. Suggestions included watching the news shows, Saturday morning cartoons as well as reading the movie reviews in the paper in order to have topics for discussion during visits or phone calls home. The age old problem of the generation gap was discussed. One man spoke of a visit with his son in which his son told him of his interest in Michael Jackson and the father spoke disapprovingly of the singer. The father worried how this might alienate his son. He was reassured by another man in the group who said that his honesty was appropriate. This man also reminded him of how the Beatles had caused disagreement between fathers and sons in a past generation. Another issue discussed was how fathers express affection to their children. The communication of loving feelings was conveyed primarily by providing material things. Men listed the toys and gifts that they would buy their children as means to express their caring. The presence of rule-making, as a somewhat rigidified way of demonstrating closeness was noted. One man stated that when his son came to visit him in the hospital he would shake hands rather than kiss him. He clarified that after a son is 13 years old a father and son shake hands instead of kiss. A particularly frightening concept for these fathers was the notion that children follow in their parents' footsteps. Men expressed their fears that they had passed some genetic anomaly or intense impulse to their children that would curse their children and doom them to a similar life. They spoke openly of wanting to shield their children from the barbed comments about mental illness made by neighborhood children and adults. They struggled with memories of times when they were poor role models and expressed the hope that their children would not completely reject them. One man said, "Even though I've done bad things I can be good." Another less hopeful statement about the future was what a father said about his place in the family, "My son the accountant, my daughter the doctor and me the bum." Fathers also wondered how much to tell their children about where they were, and at what age their child would be ready to hear about and understand their confinement. While some of the content is extreme and unique to these particular fathers and children, it is also clear that many of the themes discussed like the generation gap, passing on of unwanted traits, and communicating love, are common to many other fathers and children.

The co-leaders recognized the important therapeutic task of addressing the profound loss experienced by these men, and their inability to take part in their children's upbringing. We also helped them to consider their fears over their eventual reunion with their children.

Fathers were able to use the structure effectively. They were able to share information and feelings about each particular topic. Group leaders observed that group members were able to stay focused on the topics. One hypothesis for this might be that the issue was seen as an important component of their sense of self. While the possibility existed for these men to deny and avoid the powerful feelings associated with this role, the therapists structured the group process so that patients did not feel the need to flee from the affect. Group leaders worked to foster an atmosphere of respect, where patients could share experiences with one another and with group leaders. It was therapeutic for these men to keep contact with the outside world. They did this on behalf of their children, by staying informed about Saturday morning cartoons, news events, popular music stars and songs, current movies and the latest toys. They made this effort to maintain a sense of relationship with their children. However, it is clear that it also provided these men with a connection with the outside world.

As noted earlier, the authors observed that incarcerated fathers are an underserved treatment group. Why is this? Certainly, patients refusal to participate in treatment, the inability to identify appropriate treatment cases, and lack of available therapy resources are important factors which preclude this patient group from entering treatment. The issue of counter transference, the thoughts and feelings of the therapists, is also a factor which interferes with treatment being made available. These issues must be identified, explored and accepted before the therapy can proceed.

The authors had many questions before they began this group. They wondered what kind of role model a father could be when he has committed a crime, has been repeatedly hospitalized for mental illness or has a severe drug problem. They wondered if these children were better off with no relationship with their father. They considered ways to support and improve fathers' existing relationships with their children, and specifically how to assist a father to maintain a relationship with his child while hospitalized.

The leaders found their questions partially answered in the work, as fathers spoke movingly of their struggles in their relationships with their children.

CONCLUSION

It is clear from our work with this group that the issue of fathering for men who are mentally ill and in penal institutions is often unrecognized. We observed that a father's separation from his child is an important issue and should be addressed in treatment. It is apparent from our experience that these men can use a group focused on fathering issues. Issues involved in being a father can be seen as a powerful expression of a man's self-esteem and sense of future. This is an area where these men are motivated and willing to address difficult interpersonal issues. They look at their children and hope that they will not experience the same failure, hate, and neglect.

On inpatient wards today treatment is directed toward controlling major psychiatric symptoms, i.e., paranoid persecutory delusions, command hallucinations, and very real threats of violence directed inward and outward. These issues are extremely important and are rightly the focus of a short-term hospitalization. However, the authors suggest that the issues of fathering are important and salient ones for mentally ill men. It is the experience of the authors that the issues of fathering are available for treatment in a short-term task focused group psychotherapy.

REFERENCES

Abdullah O., Davis L., Haley J., Smith B., & Souza J. (1981). *A day in life, a day in prison* Boston, MA· Department of Mental Health.

Biller H.B. (1981) Father absence, divorce, and personality development. In M.E. Lamb (Ed.), *The role of the father in child development.* New York. John Wiley.

Fraiberg S., Adelson E., and Shapiro V. (1975). Ghosts in the nursery. *American Journal of Child Psychiatry*, 14, 387-421.

Gamer E., and Gamer C.P. (1983). *There is no solitary confinement–A look at the impact of incarceration upon the family.* Paper presented at the Association for the Professional Treatment of Offenders, Chestnut Hill, MA.

Gamer E., and Schrader A.K. (1981). Children of incarcerated parents Problems and intervention. In I. Stuart and L. Abt (Eds.), *Children of separation and divorce: Management and treatment.* New York Van Nostrand Rheinhold.

Marsh R.L. (1983). Services for families: A model project to provide services for families of prisoners. *International Journal of Offender Therapy and Comparative Criminology*, *27*, 156-162.

Raubolt R R , and Rachman A.R. (1980). A therapeutic group experience for fathers. *International Journal of Group Psychotherapy*, *30*, 229-239.

Sack W.H., Seidler J., and Thomas S. (1976). The children of imprisoned parents A psychosocial exploration. *American Journal of Orthopsychiatry*, *46*, 618-628.

An Educational Occupational Issues Group for the Chronic Psychiatric Patient

Beatrice Grillo-DiDemenico

SUMMARY. Chronic psychiatric patients often do not succeed in employment or obtaining social services because they lack the ability to understand employers and social service organizations. Serious disorders and symptomatology, as well as the lack of skills, hinder their success. An educational group can provide the knowledge needed for understanding businesses and organizations and how they involve the individual.

THE EDUCATIONAL OCCUPATIONAL ISSUES GROUP

The Continuing Services Program is a psychiatric outpatient clinic of Bayley Seton Hospital, whose services are delivered by St. Vincent's North Richmond Community Mental Health Center of Staten Island, New York. The program is modeled after the Continuing Care Clinic (C.C.C.) established in February 1969 as a unit of the outpatient clinic of Michigan Neuropsychiatric Institute and presented for consideration by Brandwin, van Houten, and Neal, in *Psychiatry* in 1976.

An Educational Occupational Issues Group was formed at the C.S.P. in order to provide chronic psychiatric patients with basic occupational precepts which were not learned through normal channels. An educational approach which analyzes businesses and organizations helps the patient understand what is expected of him/her in the capacity of a worker or as a recipient of social services. The population of C.S.P. consists of patients with primary psychotic

Beatrice Grillo-DiDemenico, ACSW-P, is Psychiatric Social Worker, St Vincents North Richmond Community Services Program of Bayley Seton Hospital, Staten Island, NY.

disorders, severe characterological disorders, and borderline conditions.

C.S.P.* is designed to serve the needs of chronically mentally ill patients who have not responded well to other treatment approaches. These chronic patients have unique personality traits that often are not compatible with the structure of existing outpatient programs. Noncompliance, due to severe impairments, is a major issue which often places the total treatment plan in jeopardy.

In order to provide appropriate treatment, a program has been established to meet the needs of this population. The clinic is available on a walk-in basis, four times a week. Scheduled appointments are limited to psychiatric evaluations provided by two psychiatrists, and a Prolixin/Haldol program is administered by two registered nurses. The walk-in patients are serviced by one of three therapists, a Ph.D., who is Director of the Program, and two Certified Social Workers, who share responsibility for treatment. Each patient is seen on a first-come basis in order of arrival time. In addition four therapeutic groups are available as part of the overall treatment process. The walk-in service fosters identification with the agency rather than with one individual therapist. It affords multiple relationships with several staff members, thereby reducing the possibility of an intense dependency relationship with one therapist; the service is also therapeutic, as these patients cannot tolerate intensity of transference. Continuity of care is guaranteed by sharing of information at staff meetings. Some patients are assigned one therapist if the staff determines that this approach would be more appropriate to the patients' needs.

Once registered with the program, the patient decides the frequency of visits within a structured time frame; he/she is not denied services because of long absences from the program or noncompliance with medication. Unless initiated by the patient, termination from the program is not anticipated, and patients who do leave are guaranteed reentry if it appears to be clinically beneficial.

During the course of providing therapy at C.S.P., I became aware of recurring themes concerning employers and employment.

*The description of C.S.P. was drawn from Phillipps, Martin J. Original Clinic/Program design Mimeographed paper. (1981).

On exploration, it became clear that many patients did not succeed in employment not only because of their serious psychiatric disorders, narcissistic qualities, and lack of skills, but also because of erroneous ideas and an absence of accurate occupational precepts. Ideally, this basic knowledge should have been obtained through parental guidance, schooling, and exchange of information with experienced workers. Lack of education in this area had led these patients in the past to make poor decisions, which resulted in failure and further reinforcement of low self-esteem.

In order to provide the information the patients are deprived of and stimulate ventilation of individual concerns, an Educational Occupational Issues Group was originated where concepts as to what makes small businesses, firms, agencies, and social services programs successful are discussed, as well as what is expected of the individual in order for these establishments to meet their goals. Programs discussed include the Social Security Administration, Department of Maintenance, Social Supplement Income, Social Security Disability, and New York State Unemployment Benefits. The purpose of the group is to provide knowledge needed to acquire and maintain employment, and not necessarily to gain employment for the patients. Appropriate interaction with various government agencies is a major topic of discussion. Members of the group are referrals from other C.S.P. centers. Each member is interviewed individually by the leader to determine whether there is an interest in the subject area, the capacity for cognitive participation, and the capacity to form relationships.

The meetings are held once a week for one hour with a group of approximately six participants. Discussion is limited to vocational and occupational issues, although often it is uncertain if topics presented are related and appropriate. On these occasions group members are asked to make a correlation. When members leave the group new individuals are recruited.

Topics discussed in the group include history and psychology of work ethics, concepts of organizations, and issues pertinent to the individual. Members experience sharing of information, role playing, empathy, and support of individual problem-solving attempts. Interest in occupational issues, establishes ties among the members through the learning process. Sample resumes are distributed to the members and act as vehicles for ventilation of anger and sadness for being mentally ill and the difficulties mental illness presents for competitiveness in the job market. Members help each other by suggesting techniques for handling time gaps and lack of experience in their resumes without disclosing their psychiatric histories. The consensus is not to reveal any psychological problems on employment applications, which might hinder acceptance for employment.

THE SIX-BOX MODEL

A cognitive framework is instituted using as a tool a simplified version of Weisbord's concepts presented in *Organizational Diagnosis* (1985), together with a version of the Six-Box Model. This model is intended to help individuals understand aspects of organizations and how they perform more efficiently, by identifying problem areas, making recommendations, and initiating procedures for remedies. The role of the worker within the organization is emphasized.

The Six-Box Model (Figure 1) describes the interrelationship of factors in organizations. An individual chart is provided for each member to help him/her conceptualize the theory to his/her personal experience. Voluntarily, members provide the name of a business, agency, or other group they are interested in analyzing because of difficulty they experienced in their interaction. Learning what went wrong helps one succeed in future endeavors. An individual chart is used for illustration and statements. Each member participates in helping the others describe what ideas go into the different boxes, their relationships to each other, and how these ideas affect them as a worker or client.

The Six-Box Model diagram is used to examine organizations and the ideas pertaining to them and also to study individuals and their unique systems. In both instances, the Model provides a guide to deciding what changes need to be made in the individual or in the organization in order to meet its goals. The boxes of the Model are as follows:

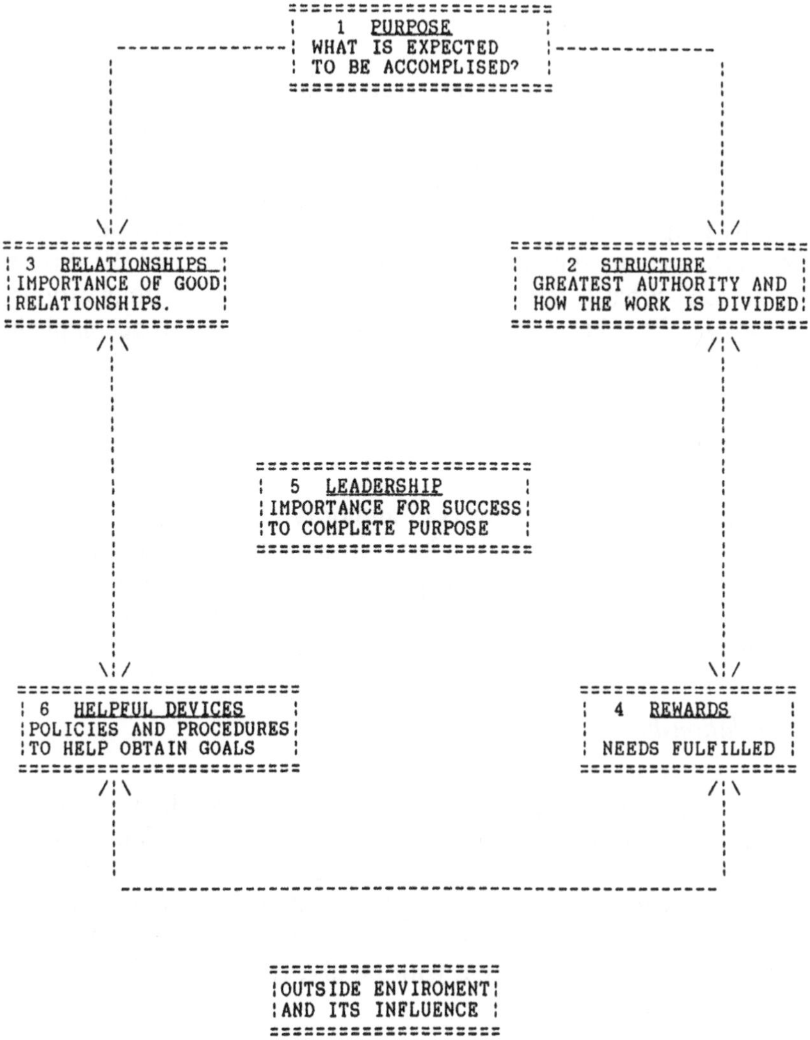

FIGURE 1 THE SIX-BOX MODEL (FROM WEISBORD, 1985, FIGURE 1, P 9)

1. Purpose

The purpose box refers to the mission of the establishment, what is expected to be accomplished. Purpose is a unique feature that differentiates the business and the worker. And the worker needs to know what the business is all about and his/her role in accomplishing the purpose. The worker must also explore the purpose of his/her participation. Why does an individual want to work? What is to be gained? What is the purpose of soliciting services from various agencies? What behaviors are beneficial in helping to accomplish the purpose.

2. Structure

Structure refers to the levels of authority in the organization and how the work is divided. Workers' responsibilities and duties are discussed in reference to the organizations being reviewed. Structure is also applied to the individual in order to ensure success in employment and everyday life.

3. Relationships

The importance of good relationships between fellow workers, supervisors, different units in the organization, and outside environment is emphasized, not only for the organization as a whole, but for the individual as well. The negative and positive effects and the consequences of interdependence are explored. Relationships in general, including interaction with family, friends, neighbors, etc. are discussed.

4. Rewards

Rewards are the method whereby the needs of the organization and/or individuals are fulfilled. Specific rewards, such as growth, self-esteem, socialization, education, creativity, financial remuneration and fringe benefits are investigated.

5. Leadership

The leader is the person or persons who keep all the elements in balance in order to maintain stability needed for the organization to accomplish its purpose. This task is important because responsibility for the success of the organization lies with management. Characteristics of good leaders and their interdependence with other workers are areas of focus and exploration. When analyzing an individual leadership represents the individual.

6. Helpful Devices

Devices* are described as aids in coordinating work, monitoring or keeping track of work, and identifying problem areas. Any policy procedure or tool, such as meetings, scheduling, and on-the-job training, that helps people work better and enables the organization or individual to obtain goals in everyday life are also included in this category.

7. Outside Environment

Outside environment and its impact on the organization and individual are reviewed. This is a major area for discussion as many members are from a low socioeconomic class that often is not supportive for advancement. Prejudices in areas of race, religion, sex, and disabilities in general are explored, together with their impact on the individual.

The Six-Box Model easily illustrates role expectations and guidelines that lead to successful performance in employment. In addition, understanding organizations and their needs, for example, requirements of government agencies, helps patients realize the steps they must follow to procure their needs.

The Occupational Issues Group has been in existence for approximately three years. With the exception of one group member, all participants are in individual therapy in addition to group therapy. Members joined the group with the expectation of correcting defi-

*Weisbord's term "mechanism" is not applied in our program in order to simplify the concept.

ciencies of structure in their personalities and occupational areas, and all have tried hard to succeed. Three of the five original members remain participants. D. has a diagnosis of Schizoid Personality and was referred to the group because of an interest in returning to work following an absence of about eight years. E. who has a diagnosis of Schizophrenia, paranoid type, was referred from a day program for preparation to joining a vocational center and/or part-time employment. A. was referred because of acute absenteeism while attending a day treatment program. At present D. is close to seeking employment and E. is leaving the day treatment program to volunteer four days a week while continuing in the group process. A. attends the group regularly, with very few absences. Lateness, however, remains a problem and is now the primary focus of treatment. Two additional members, B. and C., have acquired full-time employment and have since left the group.

A GROUP SESSION

How patients are taught to understand employers/organizations is best demonstrated by describing a particular group session. At this meeting A. told the members that he could no longer attend the day treatment program because of acute absenteeism. Following many unsuccessful attempts to rectify this situation, the program decided to refer him to the Walk-In Clinic and to the Educational Occupational Issues Group. A. stated that the absences could not be avoided because of his unique personality traits. He felt that the day program was designed to service the psychiatric patient and that the staff's expectations and demands were unrealistic.

In order to explain why A.'s encounter with this program was not favorable, it is important to first understand the dynamics of the program itself and what it hopes to accomplish. A unique feature of this approach to learning occupational issues is that the focus is knowing the employer/organization and its goals. The expectation is that the individual will help the employer achieve these goals. It is not unusual for persons even outside the psychiatric community to fail in certain positions because they do not or cannot meet the requirements of the facility.

It is assumed that A.'s behavior and its consequences caused difficulty with the inner mechanisms of the program. In order to identify which components were affected, reference is made to the Six-Box Model (Figure 1). This model, used as a tool, concretely recognizes which areas A.'s behavior affected and what action needed to be taken by the agency.

The leader began the analysis with the first component, the purpose of the agency. It was identified as providing psychiatric services to help outpatients remain in the community. Other members contributed by pointing out additional areas. A. described the structure of the day program and its staff. A. felt the program's relationship and leadership were stable and without problems. Several members identified the program's rewards as humanitarian and monetary. A. attested to the existence of policies and procedures included in the helpful devices component, which staff and patients were expected to follow as directed. Comment was also made on the negative outside influence which almost prevented the program from operating in a certain community. The treatment program had since appeased the opposition. The consensus at the end of the review was that all areas of the program were healthy, enabling the program to accomplish its goals and objectives.

The leader then asked the members to refer to the Six-Box Model diagram to interpret why the day program could not accept A.'s chronic absenteeism. One member stated that all absences affect the purpose of the program, which is to provide services. Structure and division of work could not be maintained if the amount of patients arriving for the program could not be predicted. Leadership was also an affected area because the task assigned to leadership of successfully completing the purpose could not be accomplished. If the purpose could not be achieved, there could be no rewards. Absenteeism and noncompliance with policies and regulations severely damaged this area and affected five of the other areas. The leader also pointed out that outside environmental influences could exert pressure on the program if patients in need were not serviced.

The Six-Box Model, which had previously depicted a healthy program, now illustrated a dysfunctional treatment center at risk for closure because many internal areas were experiencing difficulty. One member's chronic absenteeism seemed a relatively simple affair; however, when focus was placed on what the center hoped to accomplish, it became a major difficulty. The leader asked the members to consider the needs of employers/organizations and how their performance affects these groups.

A.'s personal functioning was also affected by his noncompliance. In order for A. to realize this the Six-Box Model was used to analyze his difficulties. A. was represented by the component leadership. A. stated his purpose was to attend the day treatment program. He, however, did not adhere to his procedures, which would have helped him achieve his goal. Lack of planned daily activity resulted in his becoming purposeless as tasks and assignments were not completed. Relationships were affected as family, friends, and staff members were disappointed in his performance. Rewards, such as increased self-esteem through accomplishments, could not be gained. As an outside influence, positive results from attending the day treatment center also were not realized. Six dynamics in A.'s personal functioning were in difficulty. A. was able to identify the problem areas presented in this concrete form and was able to decide what changes were necessary to enhance his personal functioning.

VENTILATION OF ISSUES

The Educational Occupational Issues Group also helps patients change or correct deficiencies in personality functioning by ventilation and discussion of issues. Erroneous opinions and inappropriate opinions are confronted, forcing the member to view his/her behavior from a different perspective. The following group process describes individual unique characteristics and how the group approached these difficulties.

A., a single man in his late twenties experienced occupational difficulties due to paranoia and low self-esteem. He left high school prior to graduation and had since acquired a general education diploma. He had a diagnosis of Paranoid State, unspecified, and was referred to the Occupational Issues Group because he was not able to maintain employment for any significant length of time.

B. felt that people deliberately tried to "put him down" by pointing out his errors. He also resented not being properly trained, which ensured failure. When he felt threatened owing to feelings of inadequacy, he often left a job without giving notice. The inappropriateness of this behavior was discussed and alternative methods of handling the stress were explored. At one group meeting B. told the members that his father had arranged for a position for him as a messenger for a Manhattan firm. The interview was to take place the following Tuesday. Therefore, he explained, he could not attend group process. He expressed his fears that dynamics that occurred in past employments would once again surface to embarrass him and cause him to fail. The group globalized his feelings and each member contributed to the discussion. At the end of the meeting they wished him well and told him they were anxious for his return or feedback concerning the results of his endeavor.

It was a surprise to the group when B. returned the following Tuesday instead of reporting to work. He appeared despondent as he explained that he proceeded as far as the Staten Island ferry en route to Manhattan, when he became overwhelmed with fears and had to turn back. Members empathized with him and, through questioning, learned he had not telephoned to cancel the appointment. Opinions were stated concerning the importance of a telephone call and how it related to responsibility and how others could form a negative judgment of him. D. agreed with the members but explained that fears often override reality. All concurred but felt the telephone call was a separate issue and that he should have forced himself to make it regardless of the anxiety it provoked.

One member commented that fears occur with any new endeavor and that it is inappropriate to stop trying. Another told B. that her daughter asked her to accompany her to an interview in order to lessen the anxiety. Although she was not present during the appointment, her daughter felt more confident knowing she was nearby. The members gave B. a clear message that it was impossible to gain employment without taking risks of rejection. They added it was a process from which no one was exempt. They felt that he needed more self-discipline and less impulsiveness in decision making. B. was able to accept their constructive criticism, which was presented in a nonthreatening manner.

During this group session I informed B. that I was happy that he had decided to come to the group meeting when he could not continue to his scheduled appointment. This statement was intended to convey to B. that he was unconditionally accepted by the leader and the members. This statement also provided an opportunity for the group to verbalize their support and encourage him in future endeavors. I also introduced to the group that there was a sense of caring for each other as evidenced by their empathy and concern for B.

I asked for confirmation of this statement and prompted each member to state his/her feelings. The purpose of this intervention was to further increase the cohesiveness of the members and provide B. with an opportunity to advance his self-esteem through positive feedback. It also induced members to voice their feelings to B. and to each other. At the end of the session B.'s sadness had decreased and his mood had elevated because of the support he received from the group.

Through the use of the Six-Box Model to identify problem areas, B. has initiated changes in his personal functioning. He has learned to manage and question the paranoia in order to reduce the panic. He realizes how it affected his performance and prohibited him from achieving his goal for long-term employment. Approximately four months ago, B. gained employment and has managed to maintain the position. B. is still receiving individual therapy, but there is little contact with the group.

The fifth member, C., has also gained employment within the past several months. C., a single male in his late twenties, was referred to the Occupational Issues Group by his individual therapist. Although he was an advanced student in college at the time of his entry into the group, he explained that he had problems in staying with tasks because he became bored. He hoped the group could assist him in coping with stressful situations and help him reduce burnout, which caused poor performance and low self-esteem. C. also wanted to gain knowledge of businesses and agencies so he could one day succeed in employment. His diagnosis was Mixed Personality Disorder.

At the first group meeting when C. introduced himself, he proudly boasted of his academic achievements. As he was speaking, I became aware of silence among the members. If C. was also aware of this dynamic, he indicated no cognition of it, as he continued speaking of his difficulties, his group expectations, and his future goal of employment. I waited until C. concluded his introduction and then commented on the unusual silence at this particular meeting. No one responded, so I stated that perhaps there were many feelings pertaining to the subject of higher education. This intervention was intended to induce the members to put into words their feelings concerning this new member's educational accomplishment. Once this potentially painful subject was introduced, the members were able to share information. One member said he had attended college for a short time but realized it wasn't for him. Another spoke of his nieces and nephews attending college, which he was never able to do, and others addressed the importance of their children attending college and its influence on advancement in employment. This discussion also triggered ventilation of sadness and regrets that higher education could not be a realistic goal for some members.

Toward the end of this same meeting, I commented on how the members felt when a new person came into the group and asked if this could be another cause of the silence demonstrated earlier. Individuals were able to state that they felt uncomfortable with new members and found it difficult to share information. My introduction of this dynamic was intended to act as a catalyst for the members to reflect on this uncomfortableness and correlate it to taking risks and the potential danger of feeling foolish and rejected. Members also expanded this subject area to include relationships outside the group experience.

On subsequent sessions the group discussed C.'s boredom and commented that the feeling he described as boredom could instead be depression, which consequently caused a lack of energy. They further elaborated that if depression was a dynamic, he had to force himself to complete tasks. Different techniques learned by other members to combat depression were shared and proved helpful.

Even though C. could not attend the group for several months because his school schedule conflicted with the group sessions, he maintained contact by telephone. He called regularly, asking about the members and relaying messages concerning his status. The group became a source of encouragement and approval.

When speaking of the Occupational Issues Group, he stated that it taught him responsibility and the active role he had to play to be successful. As he acquired more positive achievements in his employment, his self-esteem increased and burnout decreased. The group provided him with a message that serious illness or not, an individual can succeed; otherwise why would an occupational issues group be offered to patients with serious diagnoses? C. stated that whenever he did not feel like going to work, he remembered the purpose of the agency he works for and his responsibility to the agency and its clients.

CONCLUSION

The Educational Occupational Issues Group affords a model from which a standard can be made. The individual can measure his behaviors and decide whether they deviate from or meet the expectations of society. Through the educational process the group provides information not previously obtained through prior learning experiences. This includes the influence and experience of the leader. The group becomes a learning center projecting standards, patterns, and acceptable behavior (Hartford, 1971). Members want to succeed not only for personal gains, but to acquire respect and recognition from other members and the leader, who fully appreciate the difficulties encountered by the individual.

This type of educational group is a valuable tool in helping patients learn to interact appropriately with the environment. Clinicians must be alert to the fact that it is not always the patient's serious symptomatology which makes him/her unsuccessful, but insufficient information in desired areas of pursuit. The patient must be convinced that the clinician believes success can be achieved. The confidence that the clinician transfers makes the patient try harder.

Expectations of this group have far exceeded what was originally intended. The members have extended the original material concerning dynamics of organizations to include interactions with psychiatric services, social resource agencies, and interpersonal relationships. The cohesiveness of the group and respect from the leader move the members toward success. Implications for the future are a variety of educational issues groups to accommodate not only chronic patients, but those with all types of psychiatric conditions. The teaching concepts are versatile and can be adjusted to meet the needs of the population being serviced. This type of group can also educate the families of patients by inviting them to be participants. It can provide an awareness of the issues that patients encounter as they engage with businesses and organizations. It can also provide a means of empathy and open communication between the patient and family.

It is essential that patients be provided with as many instruments as possible for them to succeed in a sometimes hostile environment. An Educational Occupational Issues Group is one means of helping patients to reenter the mainstream of society.

REFERENCES

Brandwin, Marvin, van Houten, Wiecher H., and Neal, David L. (1976). The Continuing Care Clinic: Outpatient Treatment of the Chronically Ill. Psychiatry, Vol. 39, May. pp. 103-109.

Hartford, Margaret E. (1971). Groups in Social Work. New York. Columbia University, pp. 31-34.

Weisbord, Marvin R (1985) Organizational Diagnosis· A Workbook of Theory and Practice. Reading, Massachusetts Addison-Wesley Publishing Company, pp. 6-45.

BOOK REVIEWS

WORKING WITH WOMEN'S GROUPS, VOLUMES 1 AND 2. Louise Yolton Eberhardt. *Whole Person Press, 1987, 172 and 144 pages.*

These little handbooks with their plastic binders remind one of the Pfeiffer and Jones' *Handbooks of Structured Experiences*. . . In fact, they can be considered clones of this genre of resource (Volume 1 cites the Handbooks in its bibliography). So, if you liked those compilations of "exercises," you will love these books! That is, you will find them to be most valuable resources if you are planning to launch women's workshops, skill development, or consciousness raising groups. They will be useful if you are supervising others who offer such programs, or consulting with self-help groups that wish to pursue such a focus.

The books offer information on various content areas and interactional experiences that can be used for group work with women. The "Introduction" presents a rationale for dealing with feminist values in all-female groups, time-frames and other tips for using the exercises, plus a nice training model with the following conceptual steps: experience; identify; analyze; generalize.

There are other general guidelines: about work with groups, about evaluation, about the learning environment, and about launching groups. In addition, the reader will find a number of sample questionnaires, feedback instruments, and other examples of "practice wisdom."

Volume 1 contains 31 exercises in the areas of *Consciousness*

Raising and Self-Discovery. These are followed by designs for three workshops: *Gay Identity Workshop*, *Assertiveness Training Workshop*, and *Leadership Skills Workshop*. Volume 2 is divided into four sections: *Sexuality*, *Male/Female Identity*, *Minority Women*, and *Career Development*. There are 46 exercises in this collection. Bibliographical resources are contained in each volume.

These designs have grown out of the 20 years' involvement with women's issues and training groups conducted by Louise Eberhardt who is an experienced organization, management, and training consultant in the Baltimore, Maryland area, and former director of the Women's Center, Columbia, Md. The second volume extends the scope of volume one and contains designs contributed out of the experience of other women.

Working with Women's Groups are rich stimulants for anyone concerned with programs in this particular area. And, in fact, many of the ideas can also be generalized to other special populations. As such, they are a valuable resource for anyone wishing to review designs that have been developed out of direct practice with women's groups.

One caution here, as with any pre-packaged resource: they should not be used rigidly or with a cook-book mentality to "do things to" a group. They should suggest, not dictate. And this is what Eberhardt also emphasizes.

Ruth R. Middleman, EdD, ACSW
Professor
Raymond A. Kent School of Social Work
University of Louisville

THE HUMAN BOND. SUPPORT GROUPS & MUTUAL AID. Harry Wasserman and Holly E. Danforth. *New York: Springer Publishing Co., 1988.*

It speaks well of a book, when, upon completion the reader wishes to recommend it to colleagues. That was the experience of this reviewer after reading *The Human Bond.*

The book focusses on 2 major areas. It first provides a rationale and justification for the use of support groups and secondly offers applied theory on how to plan and lead such groups. Similarities and differences between groups for support and for psychotherapeutic purposes are noted throughout.

The book is divided into four sections, each with several chapters. The first and longest section (99 pages) "Basic Foundations For Social Support Groups," contains chapters which address an overview of theory and research on social support and support systems, a discussion of stress and its varying types and intensities and implications for the use of support groups within this context. The second section, "Working with Support Groups" (72 pages) provides guidelines for the planning and working phases of the group by applying support group theory and emphasizing the components of mutual aid. Section III (68 pages), "Examples of Professionally Led Support Groups" describes their use in the health field, with the frail elderly, in child and family practice and in mental health. The final section, IV (7 pages), "Looking Forward," does just that. In this last section, the authors recommend a reconstructed practice and education approach that would heighten the place of support groups within the social work profession and identify areas for future research on the subject. The "Support Group Planning Guide" in the appendix summarizes in outline form, the step-by-step procedures which serve as a useful guideline for practice.

A strength of this book lies in its presentation of the place of human interaction in the healing process and of the importance of emphasizing the normality rather than deviance of the human condition. In choosing this subject, the authors say they "wish to celebrate the human bond as the main source of human decency, our capacity to feel and share with others" (p. x). Wasserman and Danforth argue that the prevalence of a clinical social work practice modeled after a psychiatric, psychotherapeutic approach has resulted in a devaluation of the importance of the human environment within which individuals function and of the natural helping processes that people use spontaneously when faced with emotional stress and pain. They advocate an approach that would "diminish the social distance between workers and members" and which would recreate the constructive aspects of spontaneous human interaction within the context of the professionally led support group. They also point out that recent research and theory have strengthened the link between social support and mental health, resulting in a growing acceptance of the former as a powerful treatment concept.

Following a presentation of the advantages and disadvantages of support groups, the authors move into a more technical discussion of three categories of stress. They identify these as acute, ameliorable chronic and permanent chronic and relate these types of stress to the assessment of support group need, and in later chapters to the groups purpose, structure and content.

For the most part, the authors do well at drawing distinctions between support and therapy groups, a challenge they describe as a "delicate task," and a "fine line to walk." However, although each of these group purposes require different conceptualizations of group composition, structure, content and worker intervention, there are instances when the differences they identify are arguable. For example, in the discussion of groups phases, they assert that since, in support groups, "the essential foci involve mutual aid, support and coping with stress . . . intragroup or leader-member conflicts do not seem to be sufficiently marked to comprise a specific phase of group development" (p. 147). Yet, the literature on support and even task group experiences (including a close inspection of several of the support group articles they cite) refer to the conflict that arises when, in efforts to establish mutual trust, members exhibit challenging and angry behavior as a means of testing the limits of "acceptance" by the worker and other group members. Interpersonal conflict is also part of the natural order of human relationships and it could be a disservice to downplay its significance and value, even within the mutual aid format. Novices could be lulled into a false expectation of support groups as being "easier" to work with than other groups. The authors also assert that in groups for support and mutual aid, behavioral change must be viewed only as a secondary gain and not a primary goal. To some extent, this distinction seems artificial, since the accepted support group goal of coping more effectively and constructively with stressful situations implies modified behavior, especially in work with perpetrators of violence and with those who exhibit blatantly self-destructive behaviors. In these and other respects, that "fine line" between support and therapy groups may be even finer than the authors indicate.

In summary, this book contributes to the literature by validating, refining and advancing the humanistic ideals that lie at the root of the social work profession. It demystifies the helping process by focusing on the naturalness of people in similar trying circumstances turning to each other, and it advances the concept of "naturalness" by identifying and conceptualizing the components of it to be brought into professional practice. The "How To" chapters provide useful and practical guidelines for support group practice. The book serves as a foundation for further work by identifying questions and areas for future research and most importantly by making assertions that lead us to rethink "therapy." It is a valuable book for social work practitioners and educators.

Julianne Wayne, MSW, EdD
Associate Dean of Academic Affairs
Boston University School of Social Work

* 9 7 8 0 8 6 6 5 6 9 9 4 1 *
T - #0201 - 101024 - C0 - 229/152/8 [10] - CB - 9780866569941 - Gloss Lamination